D0918654

Mayo Clinic on Chronic Pain

David W. Swanson, M.D.

Editor-in-Chief

MASON CREST PUBLISHERS

Philadelphia, Pennsylvania

Mayo Clinic on Chronic Pain provides reliable, practical, easy-to-understand information on managing chronic pain. Much of this information comes directly from the experience of Mayo Clinic pain specialist and other health care professionals. This book supplements the advice of your personal physician, whom you should consult for individual medical problems. *Mayo Clinic on Chronic Pain* does not endorse any company or product. Mayo, Mayo Clinic and the Mayo triple-shield logo are registered marks of Mayo Foundation for Medical Education and Research.

Hardcover Library Edition Published 2002
Mason Crest Publishers
370 Reed Road
Suite 302
Broomall, PA 19008-0914
(866) MCP-BOOK (toll free)

First printing

1 2 3 4 5 6 7 8 9 10

Library of Congress Cataloging-in-Publication Data on file at the Library of Congress

ISBN 1-59084-222-7

Printed in the United States of America

89425

About Chronic Pain

Chronic pain is a leading cause of disability in the United States and one of the most common medical problems people face. Pain organizations estimate that close to 50 million Americans—perhaps even more—live with chronic pain. You, a family member or a friend may be one of them.

Chronic pain is also among the most difficult medical conditions to treat. Many factors can influence its development. Plus not everyone responds to pain, and its treatments, in the same manner.

But there is hope. Effective therapies to manage persistent pain are becoming increasingly available. Healthful changes in your lifestyle, and, if necessary, medication, can help you control your pain and lead a more active and productive life. Within these pages, you'll find practical advice you can use each day to enjoy a fuller life, despite your pain. Much of the information is what Mayo Clinic pain specialists at the Comprehensive Pain Rehabilitation Center and the Pain Clinic in Rochester, Minnesota, use day in and day out in caring for their own patients.

About Mayo Clinic

Mayo Clinic evolved gradually at the turn of the 20th century from the frontier practice of Dr. William Worrall Mayo and his two sons, William J. and Charles H. Mayo. Pressed by the exploding growth of medical knowledge and the demands of their busy surgical practice in Rochester, Minnesota, the Mayo brothers invited other physicians to join them, pioneering the group practice of medicine. Today, with more than 2,000 physicians and scientists at its three major locations in Rochester; Jacksonville, Florida; and Scottsdale, Arizona, Mayo Clinic is dedicated to providing comprehensive diagnosis, accurate answers and effective treatments for people with both common and uncommon medical conditions.

With this depth of medical knowledge, experience and expertise, Mayo Clinic occupies a unique position as a health information resource. Since 1983, Mayo Clinic has published reliable health information for millions of consumers through a variety of award-winning newsletters, books and online services. Revenue from our publishing activities supports Mayo Clinic programs, including medical education and medical research.

Preface

Y ou may have picked up this book because you have chronic pain or you know of someone who does. You also know then how difficult chronic pain can be to live with and to treat. The pain persists, despite repeated visits to doctors and a variety of methods to try to stop it.

But just because you can't make your pain go away doesn't mean you have to suffer. When given the right tools, many people find that they can still lead active and productive lives, despite their pain.

Consider this book your toolbox. In it you'll find information on a variety of behavioral and lifestyle issues, along with appropriate use of medication, for a comprehensive approach to managing chronic pain. We begin with an explanation of how pain develops and why it's so detrimental when uncontrolled. We also review some of the more common causes of chronic pain and its costly, and sometimes devastating, effects. We then devote the rest of the book to what you can do each day to control your pain. We show you how to develop personal goals, how to set up a regular exercise program and how to modify your daily routine to save energy and reduce fatigue. We provide practical strategies for reducing stress, learning to relax, overcoming anger and frustration and improving relationships. We give you information to help you recognize when medication may be beneficial and when it may cause more harm than good. Finally, we provide a guide to complementary and alternative medicine.

The book is based on the practices of Mayo Clinic physicians, psychologists, nurses, therapists and health educators who work daily with people experiencing chronic pain.

We believe that the more you know about chronic pain, and the factors that influence it, the better equipped you'll be to manage it. Along with the advice of your personal physician, this book can help you live well and enjoy life.

David W. Swanson, M.D.
Editor-in-Chief

Contents

Chapter 1	**Understanding Pain**	1
	How you feel pain	2
	Your pain response	5
	Acute vs. chronic pain	6
	What causes chronic pain?	7
	The challenges of controlling chronic pain	7
Chapter 2	**Do You Have Chronic Pain?**	9
	Arthritis	9
	Back pain	11
	Complex regional pain syndrome	13
	Endometriosis	14
	Fibromyalgia	15
	Headache	16
	Interstitial cystitis	18
	Irritable bowel syndrome	19
	Mouth, jaw and face pain	19
	Neck pain	21
	Overuse strain injuries	22
	Pelvic floor pain	22
	Peripheral neuropathy	23
	Postherpetic neuralgia	23
	Unknown causes	24
Chapter 3	**Cycles of Chronic Pain**	25
	Behavioral cycle	25
	Communicating your pain	28
	Emotional cycle	28
	Your family's responses	31
	Breaking the cycles	34
Chapter 4	**Recognizing the Costs of Chronic Pain**	35
	Physical deconditioning	35
	Loss of sleep	36

Emotional upheaval   36
Depression   37
Difficulties at work   38
Financial strain   38
Damaged relationships   39
Chemical dependency   39
Taking one step at a time   40

Chapter 5   **Taking Control of Your Pain**   41
Understanding your role   41
Finding the right doctor   42
Keeping a journal   43
Setting SMART goals   47

Chapter 6   **Getting Moving With Exercise**   53
Improving flexibility   54
Increasing aerobic capacity   58
Building strength   60
Perfecting your posture   63
Keeping your program on track   65

Chapter 7   **Finding Your Balance**   67
How does your day balance out?   68
Putting time on your side   69
Getting more organized   70
Taking everything in moderation   70
Changing how you do things   71
Moving your body wisely   72
Avoiding temperature extremes   76

Chapter 8   **Dealing With Your Emotions and Behaviors** 77
Admitting your loss   77
Managing your anger   79
Practicing positive thinking   80
Challenging your expectations   82
Learning to assert yourself   83
Boosting your self-esteem   85

Chapter 9	**Managing Life's Stresses**	87
	How you respond to stress	87
	What are your triggers?	88
	Strategies for reducing stress	89
	Relief through relaxation	91

Chapter 10	**Interacting With Family and Friends**	95
	Benefits of social interaction	95
	Developing a strong support system	96
	Improving your communication skills	97
	Ways family and friends can help	98

Chapter 11	**Caring for Yourself and Your Health**	101
	Getting a good night's sleep	101
	Controlling your weight	104
	Eating for better health	108
	Limiting alcohol	111
	Quitting smoking	112
	Expressing your sexuality	114
	Addressing your spiritual needs	117

Chapter 12	**What About Medication?**	119
	Simple pain relievers	119
	Potent painkillers	122
	Other pain medications	125
	Medications for associated conditions	126
	Injections	130
	The medication crutch	132

Chapter 13	**Complementary and Alternative Medicine**	133
	The mind and body connection	134
	Healing through manipulation and touch	136
	Restoring natural energy forces	139
	Homeopathic and naturopathic medicine	142
	How to approach nontraditional therapies	144

Chapter 14   **Pain Centers and Clinics**   145
               Types of pain programs   145
               The pain team   146
               What to expect   147
               How to locate a pain facility   148
               What to look for   148
               Your role   150

Chapter 15   **How to Stay in Control**   151
               10 ways to maintain your gains   151
               Getting through a difficult day   154
               Joining a support group   155
               It's up to you   156

Your Personal Planner   *157*

Additional Resources   *167*

Index   *171*

Chapter 1

Understanding Pain

*P*ain is universal. You can trace its trail through time—from a toothache evident in fossil remains of a human jawbone to today's drugstore shelves stacked with pain relievers. Almost half of all Americans seek treatment for pain each year, 7 million from newly diagnosed back pain alone.

Pain is also complex. There are times when it's beneficial, such as when you grasp a hot iron skillet with a bare hand or stub your toe on an oak dresser at full stride. Like a blaring alarm, pain screams its urgent warning that something is terribly wrong. But other pain—the day-after-day ache of arthritis or constant throbbing of a headache— serves no useful purpose. And its relentlessness can be overwhelming.

Above all, pain is unique. The discomfort it can cause is as varied as those who experience it. Your degree of pain and how you react to it are the results of your own biological, psychological and cultural makeup.

These insights into the many components involved in the pain process are improving people's understanding of pain and its treatment.

No longer is pain viewed as just a symptom of another disease. It can become an illness unto itself. Strategies on how best to manage pain are also evolving. For persistent pain, called chronic pain, medication alone often isn't the best form of treatment. A comprehensive approach that includes exercise, relaxation skills and behavioral changes can help control pain, but without risk of serious side effects.

Unfortunately, there often is no cure for chronic pain. And, like many other people, you may have to cope with this problem the rest of your life. But the good news is that, despite having chronic pain, you can still live an active and productive life.

This book can help you not only better understand your pain and its harmful effects, but more importantly, explain how you can take control of your pain—instead of letting *it* control *you*.

How you feel pain

Understanding how your body feels pain will help you appreciate how unique your pain experiences are. It will also help you better understand why chronic pain is often difficult to treat.

Pain basically results from a series of electrical and chemical exchanges involving three major components: your peripheral nerves, spinal cord and brain.

Your peripheral nerves

Your peripheral (puh-RIF-uh-rul) nerves encompass a network of nerve fibers that branch throughout your body, including your hands and feet. Attached to some of these fibers are special nerve endings that can "sense" an unpleasant stimulus, such as a cut, burn or painful pressure. These nerve endings are called nociceptors (NO-si-SEP-turs).

You have millions of nociceptors in your skin, bones, joints, muscles and the protective membrane around your internal organs. (You can't feel pain in your internal organs themselves.)

Nociceptors are concentrated in areas more prone to injury, such as your fingers and toes. That's why a splinter in your finger hurts more than one in your stomach or shoulder. There may be as many as 1,300 nociceptors in just 1 square inch of skin.

3. Your brain interprets the messages as pain, including its location, intensity and nature (burning, aching, stinging)

2. Pain messages move through nerves up the spinal cord

1. Pain source

Making sense of your nervous system

Your nervous system is composed of strands of nerve cells that transmit and receive messages in the form of electrical currents. It's through this intricate web of cells that your body and brain communicate.

Two main systems make up your nervous system: your central nervous system, which includes your brain and spinal cord, and your peripheral nervous system. Your peripheral nerves extend from your spinal cord to your skin, muscles and internal organs. Within each of these systems are three major categories of nerves:

- Autonomic nerves maintain normal body processes, such as breathing, heart rate, blood pressure, digestion, perspiration and sexual function.
- Motor nerves are responsible for movement of your muscles. They allow you to move your hands and feet, walk or sit.
- Sensory nerves are your "sensing" nerves. They allow you to feel an object when you touch it. They're also the nerves that allow you to feel pain.

Muscles, protected beneath your skin, have fewer nerve endings. And organ membranes, protected by skin, muscle and bone, have fewer still.

Some nociceptors sense sharp blows, others heat. One type senses pressure, temperature and chemical changes. Nociceptors also can detect inflammation caused by injury, disease or infection.

When nociceptors detect a harmful stimulus, they relay their pain messages in the form of electrical impulses along a peripheral nerve to your spinal cord and brain. However, the speed by which the messages travel can vary. Dull, aching pain—such as an upset stomach or an ear-ache—is relayed on fibers that travel at a slow speed. Sensations of severe pain are transmitted almost instantaneously.

Your spinal cord

When pain messages reach your spinal cord, they meet up with special-ized nerve cells that act as "gatekeepers," allowing or refusing the mes-sages to pass through to your brain.

For severe pain that's linked to a danger, such as when you touch a hot stove, the "gate" is wide open and the messages take an express route to your brain. Nerve cells in your spinal cord also respond to these urgent warnings by triggering other nervous systems into action, such as your motor nerves. Your motor nerves signal your muscles to pull your hand away from the burner. Weak pain messages, however, such as from a scratch, may be refused entry through the "gate."

Within your spinal cord, the messages also can change. Other sensations may overpower and diminish the pain messages. This happens when you massage or apply pressure to the injured area. The result is that the warnings sent by your peripheral nerves are downgraded to a lower priority.

Nerve cells in your spinal cord also may release chemicals that amplify or subdue the messages, affecting the speed at which they travel to your brain (see "Natural painkillers and pain-enhancers").

Your brain

Once pain messages reach your brain, they arrive at the thalamus (THAL-uh-mus), a sorting and switching station located deep inside your brain. The thalamus quickly interprets the messages as pain and

---

Natural painkillers and pain-enhancers

Your brain and spinal cord produce their own painkillers that are similar to the narcotic drug morphine, used to treat severe pain. Two of these morphine-like pain relievers are called endorphins (en-DOR-fins) and enkephalins (en-KEF-uh-lins). When released, these substances attach to special receptors in your brain, producing "stop-pain" messages.

Other substances in your body do just the opposite. They intensify your pain. A protein called substance P stimulates nerve endings at the injury site and within your spinal cord, increasing pain messages. Other pain-enhancers work by activating normally silent nerve cells in the injured area. The activation prompts the cells to discharge pain messages even when the stimulation they detect isn't painful. This not only worsens the pain but also enlarges the area of sensitivity.

forwards them simultaneously to the thinking part of your brain, called the cerebral (suh-REE-brul) cortex, and to your brain's limbic center. The limbic center produces emotions such as anxiety, fear or frustration that often accompany pain. It's at this point that you actually begin to feel the pain.

Your cerebral cortex reacts to the pain messages by locating the source of the injury, assessing the damage and determining a course of action, such as ordering you to take pressure off your foot if you've sprained your ankle.

The cerebral cortex also relays additional key messages. For instance, if you've cut your finger, it signals your autonomic nervous system, the system that controls your blood flow, to send additional blood and nutrients to the injury site. It also dispatches the release of pain-suppressing chemicals and sends "stop-pain" messages back to the injury site. This alerts the nociceptors that their signals have been received.

Your pain response

When pain messages reach your brain, two components determine how you respond to the pain.

Physical sensation
Pain comes in many forms: sharp, jabbing, throbbing, burning, stinging, tingling, nagging, dull and aching. Sharp and jabbing pain generally produces greater discomfort than dull, aching pain. It's also more likely to make you anxious or fearful.

Pain also varies from mild to severe. Severe pain grabs your attention more quickly and generally produces a greater physical and emotional response than mild pain. Severe pain also can incapacitate you, making it difficult or impossible to sit or stand.

The location of your pain also can affect your response to it. A headache that interferes with your ability to work or concentrate may be more bothersome, and therefore receive a stronger response, than arthritic pain in your knee or a cut to your finger.

Personal makeup
Your emotional and psychological state, memory of past pain experiences, upbringing and attitude also affect how you interpret pain messages and tolerate pain.

For example, a minor sensation that would barely register as pain, such as a dentist's probe, can actually produce exaggerated pain for a child who's never been to the dentist and who's heard horror stories of what it's like.

But your emotional state also can work in your favor, reducing even major pain messages. This was illustrated in a pain study that compared formerly wounded war veterans with men in the general population. Men in both groups had the same kind of surgery. The combat veterans, however, required less pain medication than the others, perhaps because they thought that the surgery was a minor matter compared with what they had experienced in battle.

Athletes also can condition themselves to endure pain that would incapacitate others. In addition, if you're brought up in a home or a culture that teaches "grin and bear it," "no pain, no gain" or "bite the bullet," you may experience less discomfort than people who focus on their pain or are more prone to complain.

Acute vs. chronic pain

Acute pain is triggered by tissue damage. It's the type of pain that generally accompanies illness, an injury or surgery.

Acute pain may be mild and last just a moment, such as from a sting. Or it can be severe and last for weeks or months, such as from a burn, pulled muscle or broken bone.

When you have acute pain, you know exactly where it hurts. In fact, the word acute comes from the Latin word for "needle," referring to a sharp pain. A toothache from a cavity, a burning elbow from a scrape and abdominal pain from surgery are examples of acute pain. In a fairly predictable period, the pain generally fades away—when the cavity is filled, the skin grows back or the incision heals.

Chronic pain hangs on after the injury is healed—generally for 6 months or longer. This is reflected in the word itself: Chronic comes from the Greek word for "time."

As with acute pain, chronic pain spans the full range of sensations and intensity. It can feel tingling, jolting, burning, dull or sharp. The pain may remain constant or it can come and go, like a migraine that develops without warning.

Unlike acute pain, however, with chronic pain you may not know the reason for the pain. The original injury shows every indication of being healed, yet the pain remains—and may be even more intense.

Chronic pain also can occur without any indication of injury. Years ago, people who complained of pain that had no apparent cause were thought to be imagining the misery or trying to get attention. Doctors now know that's not true. Chronic pain is real.

What causes chronic pain?

Frequently, the cause of chronic pain is unknown. There isn't any evidence of disease or damage to your body tissues that doctors can link to the pain.

Sometimes, chronic pain is due to a chronic condition, such as arthritis, that produces painful inflammation in your joints, or fibromyalgia, that causes aching in your muscles.

Occasionally, chronic pain may stem from an accident, infection or surgery that damages a peripheral or spinal nerve. This type of nerve pain that lingers after the original injury heals is called neuropathic (NEUR-o-PATH-ik)—meaning the damaged nerve, not the original injury, is causing the pain. Neuropathic pain also can result from diseases such as diabetes or alcoholism.

Once damaged, the nerve may send pain messages that are unwarranted. For example, an increased blood sugar level associated with diabetes can damage the small nerves in your hands and feet, leaving you with a painful burning sensation in your fingers and toes.

Mystery shrouds many of the reasons why injured nerves sometimes misfire and send wrong messages. However, one reason is that when a nerve cell is destroyed, the severed end of the surviving fiber can sprout a tangle of unorganized nerve fibers (neuroma). This bundle of nerve tissue then starts sending warnings of injuries that don't exist. The unorganized fibers also refuse to follow normal checks and balances that control the rest of your nervous system, keeping pain at bay.

The challenges of controlling chronic pain

Chronic pain is common. It's estimated that almost half of Americans experience some form of chronic pain during their lifetime. But coping with the pain is often frustrating.

Pain is a very personal experience. No one except you can completely understand what you're feeling. Persistent pain can also be difficult to treat. Occasionally, surgery can cure or reduce it. And for some types of chronic pain, medication or injections are beneficial. Frequently, though, none of these approaches is effective. The pain lingers, despite repeated trips to doctors and various efforts to stop it.

However, that doesn't mean there isn't any hope. You may not be able to make your pain disappear. But you can learn how to manage the pain and improve your quality of life.

Living well despite chronic pain has a lot to do with your attitude and lifestyle. Your attitude affects your pain, for better or worse. If you have a negative attitude and view yourself as a victim of your pain, your pain will continue to control your life and consume all of your energy. It's people who are able to approach their condition with a positive attitude and a willingness to change who are often the most successful in coping with their pain.

Your lifestyle also has a significant effect on your pain. Many things you do during your day—or don't do—can intensify your pain. Identifying those factors that add to your discomfort and learning how to change them will help you keep your pain within a tolerable level.

Key steps to help you live better with chronic pain may include:
- Weaning yourself from unnecessary medications
- Becoming more physically active
- Organizing your day and performing daily tasks more efficiently
- Practicing techniques that relieve stress and promote relaxation
- Identifying your capabilities, not just your limitations
- Understanding and expressing the feelings pain creates
- Improving communication with family members and friends
- Practicing good health habits, including following a nutritious diet, managing your weight and getting adequate sleep

This book can help you seek out factors that may be contributing to your pain. It also includes strategies and suggestions for how to make positive life changes. With your doctor and other health care profes- sionals, plus your family and friends, you can learn a new way to live that takes you beyond your pain.

Chapter 2

Do You Have Chronic Pain?

Chronic pain can strike just about any part of your body, from your head to your toes, from your skin to your well-protected internal organs. Arthritis, back pain and headache are the most common types of chronic pain. But chronic pain can occur in many forms and for many reasons. Your pain may be related to an existing illness or stem from an accident or injury. Perhaps your pain is linked to a condition that doctors don't fully understand. Or maybe it has no apparent cause. In this chapter, we take a look at some of the more common types of chronic pain and why they occur.

Arthritis

Arthritis means joint inflammation. Although people often talk about it as one disease, it's not. There are many forms of arthritis. Some forms appear gradually. Others suddenly appear and then disappear, only to return again later. The disease can strike any joint in your body and may be triggered by various causes, including an injury, lack of physical activity, natural wear on your joints and genetic disease. The two most common forms of arthritis are osteoarthritis and rheumatoid arthritis.

Osteoarthritis

It makes up about half of all arthritis and affects close to 20 million Americans. This common condition results when cartilage that cushions the ends of bones in your joints starts to deteriorate. If the cartilage wears down completely, you may be left with bone rubbing against bone, inflaming the joint and producing pain.

Your body tries to repair the damage, but often the repairs are unsuccessful, resulting in growth of new bone along the sides of existing bone. The new bone may produce bony lumps, most noticeably in your hands and feet, and especially at the middle joints or ends of your fingers and toes. These lumps, called spurs, may or may not produce pain and tenderness.

Osteoarthritis most often develops after age 45 and occurs equally in men and women. It can develop anywhere in your body, but it tends to be most common in your hands and feet and in major joints in your neck, back, knees and hips. The disease generally is associated with years of wear on your joints. But the damage may be related to an imbalance of enzymes in a joint, which causes cartilage to break down faster than it's rebuilt.

Initially, arthritis pain may be minor and hurt only when you use the affected joint. But in time, the pain can intensify and hurt even when you're not using the joint.

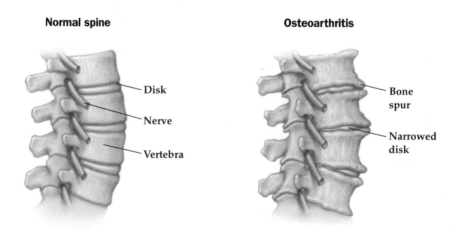

Normal spine

Disk

Nerve

Vertebra

Osteoarthritis

Bone spur

Narrowed disk

Elastic structures called disks cushion vertebrae in a normal spine, keeping it flexible. In osteoarthritis, disks narrow, leading to bony lumps along the sides of bones. Pain and stiffness may occur where bone surfaces rub together.

Rheumatoid arthritis

Unlike osteoarthritis, rheumatoid arthritis likely stems from
an immune system disorder
that causes your immune system
to attack the lining in your
joints, just as it does intruding
viruses or bacteria.

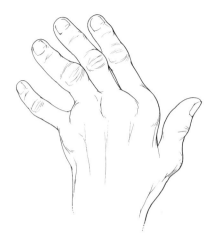

White blood cells designed
to destroy viruses and bacteria
move into joint tissues, producing inflammation and pain.
Swelling of the tissues triggers
the release of natural chemicals
that eventually dissolve cartilage and damage tendons and
ligaments in the joint.

**Rheumatoid arthritis often leads to a deformity
in fingers. During flare-ups of your disease, your
hand may be painful and weak.**

Gradually, the joint loses its
shape. In some cases, the disease destroys the joint.

Rheumatoid arthritis most often affects joints in your wrists, hands,
feet and ankles. It also can invade your elbows, shoulders, hips, knees,
neck and jaw. In addition to pain and swelling, you may experience
stiffness and loss of motion in the joints.

The disease typically develops between ages 20 and 50. An estimated 2 million Americans have rheumatoid arthritis, and roughly twice as
many women as men are affected by it.

Back pain

Back pain ranks second only to headaches as the most frequent cause of
pain. Four of five adults, at some time in their lives, experience a bout
of back pain that causes them to see a doctor.

Most back pain occurs in your lower back (lumbar area), which bears
most of your weight. Your lower back also serves as your body's pivot
point, allowing you to bend forward and backward and twist sideways.

Acute back pain often stems from an injury or accident and has a
known origin. But what causes some people to experience lingering
back pain is less clear. The pain may be related to one of the following
conditions:

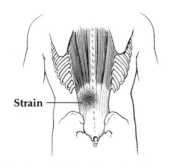

Strain —

Your lower back, a pivot point for turning at your waist, is vulnerable to muscle strains.

Muscle strain and spasm

Muscle strain is a common cause of back pain. It can occur if you lift something too heavy, twist too sharply or stand on your feet too many hours. Muscle spasm also may occur. Spasm is your back's response to injury, designed to immobilize you and prevent further damage. Any movement of the injured muscles can set off a wave of stabbing pains.

The good news is that about 90 percent of these strains heal within 4 weeks, usually much sooner. The remaining 10 percent take longer to heal. In some cases, the pain never goes away and becomes a chronic problem.

Sciatica

This condition is named for (si-AT-ik) nerve that extends leg from your buttock to you Nerve inflammation or com nerve root in your lower bac sciatica. You may feel the pa ing from your back down th your buttock to your lower l Tingling, numbness or musc weakness also can occur.

Usually, the pain resolves on its own. However, severe nerve compression can cause pro-gressive muscle weakness ar continued pain.

Sciatica is pain that radiates from your back down your buttock to your lower leg. It may be caused by inflamma-tion or compression of the roots of your sciatic nerve.

Sciatic nerve

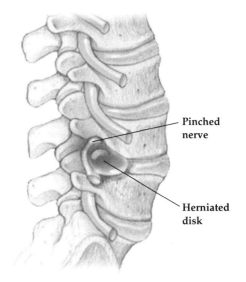

Wear and tear or injury can cause disks to rupture (herniate), creating painful pressure on nerves.

Pinched nerve

Herniated disk

Herniated disk

Normal wear and tear or strain can cause a disk between the bones in your back (vertebrae) to bulge or rupture (sometimes called a "slipped disk"). When the disk ruptures, the jelly-like interior of the disk pokes out from its normal position between your vertebrae.

Many people have damaged disks and aren't bothered by them. But if the bulging material presses against an adjacent nerve, the condition may become painful.

Generally, the rupture heals over time and the pain goes away. But in some cases, the pain can persist.

Additional causes

Other conditions that may also lead to chronic back pain include:
- Joint degeneration from arthritis
- Loss of bone mass due to osteoporosis
- Reduced muscle tone caused by physical inactivity

Complex regional pain syndrome

A bug bite can set this pain off. So can a broken bone, sprain, surgical incision or any number of other injuries—usually to your hand or foot. Before long, you're experiencing a bewildering variety of painful symptoms not only at the injury site but also beyond it.

This condition used to be known as reflex sympathetic dystrophy because it was thought to stem from an overreaction of your sympathetic nervous system, part of your autonomic nervous system that controls your heart rate, blood pressure and skin temperature. But now, doctors are unsure of its cause. In fact, complex regional pain syndrome—often called CRPS—is one of the least understood forms of chronic pain.

The condition is difficult to diagnose because it's similar to other nerve-related conditions. However, it typically includes these unique characteristics:

- Pain that lasts longer and more intensely than you would expect from the injury
- Blood flow changes to skin in the affected area, altering its temperature and color
- Abnormal hair growth on the affected limb

In most cases the pain persists for more than 6 months, and in about 25 percent of the cases, for a year or more.

Endometriosis

Endometriosis results when pieces of the lining of a woman's uterus (endometrium) migrate out of the uterus through the fallopian tubes. These pieces plant themselves on other pelvic organs, such as the pelvic walls and the outer walls of the ovaries or fallopian tubes.

Some women with endometriosis experience no pain, but others have frequent pain. The pain may be steady or it may come and go. Often, the pain is described as pressurelike aching in the lower abdomen, back and rectum that may radiate into the vagina, nearby muscles and thighs.

Other symptoms may include:

- Intense cramping during menstrual periods and pain that extends a week before and after each period
- Deep pelvic pain during intercourse
- Pain during bowel movements or urination

Endometriosis generally doesn't develop until after the onset of menstruation and rarely occurs after menopause. In some women, the condition gets worse with time.

Fibromyalgia

Fibromyalgia is a disorder that targets your muscles, tendons and ligaments. It differs from arthritis in that the pain is in nearby joint tissues instead of the joints themselves. Also unlike arthritis, it doesn't cause inflammation—just pain.

The main symptom of fibromyalgia is an "aching all over." The pain may be a deep ache or a burning sensation. Other symptoms associated with fibromyalgia may include:
- Chronic fatigue
- Difficulty sleeping
- Stiffness
- Headaches
- Pain during menstruation
- Digestive problems
- Numbness
- Tingling
- Sensitivity to weather and temperature changes

Because its symptoms are many and varied and they don't follow a consistent pattern, fibromyalgia is often called fibromyalgia syndrome.

Most often, symptoms of fibromyalgia first become noticeable in your 30s. They may flare and then subside, but they usually don't disappear completely. Although fibromyalgia tends to stay with you, it isn't progressive, crippling or life-threatening.

Doctors aren't sure what causes this condition. One theory is that certain factors, such as stress, poor sleep, physical or emotional trauma or being out-of-shape, may trigger the condition in people who are more sensitive to pain. Numerous other possibilities as to its cause also are under study.

Doctors generally diagnose fibromyalgia only after they've tested for and eliminated the possibility of other conditions.

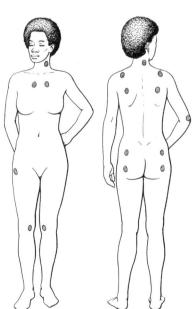

Common locations of painful aching associated with fibromyalgia.

Headache

Of all the pains people experience, headache is the most widespread complaint. Nearly everyone gets a headache at one time or another.

Headaches can range from fleeting annoyances to those that lay you flat on your back for days and return often enough that they become a chronic problem.

There are several types of headaches. Most fall into one of the three following categories:

Tension-type

These make up 9 of 10 headaches. They range from mild to severe, and they can disrupt your daily routine in varying degrees. You may experience a slow-building, dull, tight, pressurized pain that envelops your forehead, scalp, back of the neck or both sides of your head. Occasionally the pain may be burning or throbbing.

Many cases of tension-type headache appear to result from contraction of the muscles on the outside of your skull. There's some evidence that enlargement of blood vessels in your scalp also may contribute to the pain. Tension-type headaches are often triggered by stressful events such as a demanding job, a bumper-to-bumper commute or an argument with a friend or family member. Staring at a computer all day also can produce tension-type headaches. If the tension persists, the headaches can become a chronic problem.

Migraine

More than 20 million Americans experience a more painful variety of headache known as migraine. This type of headache not only gets your attention but also can put your life on hold.

Migraines generally produce throbbing pain on one side of your head—often your temple or forehead. Bright lights and loud noises may intensify the pain, and you may become nauseated and vomit. The pain can range from moderate to severe. Most migraines linger for only a few hours before peaking and slowly subsiding.

Migraines were once thought to be chiefly related to blood circulation. During a migraine, blood vessels in your brain, neck and scalp tighten, reducing blood to your brain. This tightening is followed by a sudden expansion of the vessels to larger than their normal size, causing blood to rush into them, producing swelling and pain.

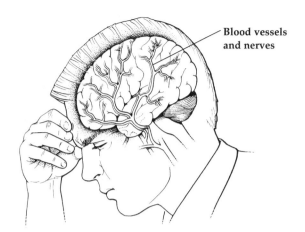

Blood vessels
and nerves

Migraines appear to stem from
an imbalance of brain chemicals which causes blood vessels in your brain to swell and
signal pain.

Researchers now believe these changes are a result of, and not the
cause of, a migraine. A more likely cause is an imbalance of brain chemicals. Several chemicals may be related in some way to development of
migraines, including the brain chemical serotonin (SER-o-TOE-nin).
During a headache, serotonin levels generally drop.

About 10 percent of people with recurrent migraines get warning
signs of an impending headache. These signals, called auras, often
involve tingling sensations or visual distortions, such as blurred vision
or zigzagging lights. They generally last less than an hour.

Migraines appear to be hereditary. They also may be triggered
by several factors:

Hormone fluctuations. Three times more women are affected by
migraines than men. About 65 percent of women who get migraines
say they occur immediately before, during or right after their period.
Estrogen found in birth control pills and in hormone replacement
therapy also may trigger migraines in some women. For other women,
their migraines diminish when taking estrogen.

Diet. Between 8 percent and 25 percent of people with migraines
point to a particular food as a source of their attacks. The most common
culprits are alcohol (especially red wine and beer), aged cheeses, choco-
late, caffeine, monosodium glutamate (MSG) and fermented, pickled or
marinated foods.

Environment. Many people cite bright light, strong odors or
changes in weather conditions as a precursor to a migraine.

Lifestyle. Daily stress can trigger a migraine. Migraines also may result from poor sleep patterns, extreme fatigue and skipping meals.

Medications. Several medications may trigger a migraine in people who are susceptible to the headaches. They include certain high blood pressure medications, some diuretic and asthma medications, birth control pills and hormone replacement therapy. Frequent use of pain medications can also produce migraines. Migraines that stem from overuse of pain medications are known as rebound headaches (see Chapter 12, page 123).

Cluster

A cluster headache is a rare but intense headache—worse than a severe migraine and one of the most excruciating head pains imaginable. It feels like a hot poker being stabbed into your eye or a drill bit boring into your skull. The pain site is usually on one side of your head, often in or around an eye or near the middle of your face by your teeth. Lying down typically worsens the pain.

Other symptoms of cluster headache can include a runny nose, red and watery eyes or a sweaty face along with a droopy eyelid.

The term cluster is used because the headaches occur in clusters over several days or weeks, then usually disappear for several months before coming back again. When the headaches strike, they often do so at the same time each day, and often at night. Generally, the headaches are short in duration, lasting 30 to 90 minutes.

Approximately 9 of 10 people who get cluster headaches are men, especially heavy smokers and heavy drinkers. Some cluster headaches also seem to be linked to seasonal changes in the amount of daylight.

Because cluster headaches are uncommon, they're sometimes misdiagnosed. They can be mistaken for a severe migraine, a sinus infection or even a dental problem because the pain may occur near your mouth.

Interstitial cystitis

This painful bladder condition affects mainly women. It results from chronic inflammation of your bladder wall. However, what causes it to develop is unknown.

Symptoms include pressure, pain and tenderness around the bladder, in addition to reduced bladder capacity, a frequent need to urinate and backaches. In some people, the pain can be so severe they have trouble riding in a car or even sitting at a desk.

The condition often mimics symptoms of a urinary tract infection, but urine tests don't detect any bacteria and antibiotics don't relieve the pain.

Irritable bowel syndrome

Irritable bowel syndrome is a complex disorder in your lower intestinal tract that causes pain, bloating, gas and recurrent bouts of diarrhea or constipation. It's a common gastrointestinal disorder and a frequent reason people see a doctor.

The pain accompanying this condition often occurs below the navel and can be dull and aching or sharp and sudden. The condition may stem from changes in the nerves that control sensation or muscle contractions in your bowel. Your central nervous system or hormonal changes also may play a role. Hormone fluctuations help explain why some women's symptoms are worse before or during menstruation.

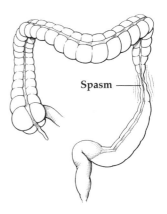

Some evidence shows that people with irritable bowel syndrome have bowels that react more strongly to stress, activity or diet than in people without the condition.

A spasm in the bowel wall may cause abdominal pain and other unpleasant symptoms commonly associated with irritable bowel syndrome.

There's little evidence that irritable bowel syndrome results from particular foods. However, in some cases, fatty foods, beans and other gas-producing foods, alcohol, caffeine and excess fiber may make symptoms worse.

Mouth, jaw and face pain

Some people experience chronic pain in their mouth, jaws and face (orofacial pain). Often, this pain is the result of dental problems, such as cavities or gum disease. But sometimes it can stem from other orofacial conditions.

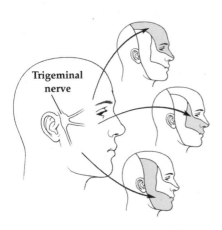

If you have trigeminal neuralgia, pain may occur in areas supplied by one of the three branches of the trigeminal (fifth cranial) nerve.

Trigeminal neuralgia

Also known as tic douloureux (doo-loo-ROO), this pain typically results when a blood vessel comes in contact with the trigeminal (tri-JEM-ih-nul) nerve, putting pressure on the nerve. The trigeminal nerve branches throughout your face and controls facial sensations and some muscles involved in chewing.

The result is an electric shock-like pain on one side of your face. It's sudden and strong enough to make you snap your head back as though you've been clubbed. Jolts of pain may persist for a few seconds to several minutes, usually returning many times a day.

For some people, even the slightest touch can trigger the pain: shaving, stroking your face, eating, talking, a slight breeze or walking into an air-conditioned room.

Temporomandibular joint disorders

The temporomandibular joints, located on each side of your face, connect your jaw to your skull. Temporomandibular joint disorders refer to a group of symptoms affecting these joints and their attached muscles. A common symptom is pain in your face, neck or ears. Other symptoms may include headaches, jaw locking or catching, and pops or clicks in your jaw during normal use.

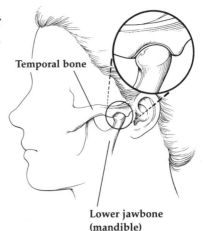

Temporal bone

Your temporomandibular joint is a hinged joint situated on each side of your head where the lower jawbone (mandible) connects with the temporal bone of your skull. Inflammation, injury or dislocation of this joint may cause pain.

Lower jawbone (mandible)

There are several theories regarding the causes of these disorders. They include trauma to the joints, degeneration of the joints and perhaps even the influence of hormones.

Other causes

Orofacial pain also can occur for other reasons that aren't well understood—and that are difficult to diagnose. Many times, the pain develops after dental treatment or a facial injury. It may be a constant aching or burning. Or, it may come in the form of frequent shocks. Nerve damage in a tooth and damage to nerves in your face are possible causes.

Neck pain

Similar to back pain, an injury or poor posture can strain muscles, ligaments or tendons in your neck, producing inflammation and pain. Most of the time the pain lasts for just a few days or weeks. Occasionally, it can become chronic.

Neck pain also may stem from a herniated disk or degeneration of joints in your upper spine as a result of osteoarthritis or loss of bone mass (osteoporosis). Instead of sliding across each other smoothly, bony surfaces in your neck impinge on each other, causing stiffness and pain.

Often, one pain leads to another. You automatically tense your neck muscles to prevent further movement in a sore spot. The tension produces pain, and may also trigger painful spasm.

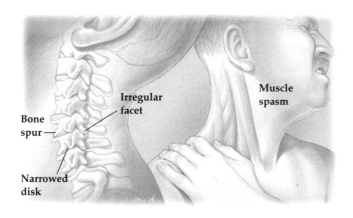

Bone spur

Irregular facet

Narrowed disk

Muscle spasm

Disks between bones in your neck can thin and lose elasticity. Bony outgrowths (spurs) may form. As joints rub together with greater-than-normal force, surfaces where they meet (facets) become irregular. Pain may result.

Overuse strain injuries

These injuries result from overuse of your muscles and tendons—mainly those in your hands, wrists and arms. The most noticeable symptom is pain. But an overuse injury also can cause tingling, weakness, numbness, swelling and stiffness.

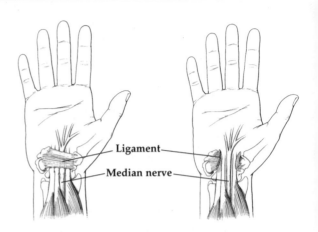

A narrow tunnel through your wrist (the carpal tunnel) protects your median nerve, which provides sensation to your fingers. When swelling occurs in the tunnel, the median nerve can become compressed, producing pain.

Computer users, assembly-line employees and meat cutters are among those most commonly affected by an overuse injury. But it can occur in anyone who uses repeated motions in their daily activities.

Carpal tunnel syndrome is the most recognized overuse injury. It results from constant strain on your wrist, which can inflame the tendons below your carpal ligament, the ligament that stretches across the palm-side of your wrist. When the tendons swell, they press against a nearby nerve located beneath your carpal ligament, producing pain. Because the nerve runs up your arm all the way to your neck, you might feel pain anywhere along that pathway.

Most often, the result is numbness, tingling or pain starting in your wrist and moving down into your thumb and first three fingers. Some people find their symptoms are worse at night because of the position of their wrist or arm while sleeping. The position of your wrists when holding a book or driving a car also may intensify the pain.

Pelvic floor pain

Your pelvic floor muscles are those muscles located at the bottom of your pelvis, between your legs. They loop around your rectum and attach to the front of your pelvis. The muscles help you eliminate body wastes. But if they work improperly, they may cause recurrent pain.

In some cases, the pain may result from intense muscle spasm. Other times, the muscles don't relax as they normally should during a bowel movement. Instead, they contract even tighter, causing constipation and pain. The cause of these muscle disorders is often unknown.

Peripheral neuropathy

This nerve-related condition most often affects your hands and feet, causing a tingling pain that's generally accompanied by numbness. In some cases, the pain also can be shooting or burning.

Peripheral neuropathy can result from many causes, including side effects of medication, infection or vitamin deficiencies. The most common causes are diabetes, alcoholism and autoimmune diseases (such as rheumatoid arthritis or lupus) that can damage small nerve endings. There are also times when the cause of peripheral neuropathy is unclear.

The condition usually starts with a tingling sensation in your toes or the balls of your feet which spreads upward. Occasionally, it begins in your hands and extends up your arms. Numbness may follow and proceed in the same manner. Your skin also may become highly sensitive, with even the slightest touch triggering pain.

Postherpetic neuralgia

Postherpetic neuralgia (POST-her-PET-ik neu-RAL-juh) refers to nerve damage that occurs as a result of shingles, a viral infection. The damaged fibers aren't able to send normal pain messages. Instead, the messages become distorted and exaggerated, producing unrelenting, and often severe, pain.

Pain associated with this condition can take different forms: burning, sharp and jabbing or

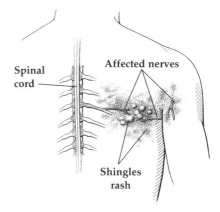

Shingles rash is associated with an inflammation of nerves beneath the skin. Damage to the nerves may produce postherpetic neuralgia.

deep and aching. Your skin also may become hypersensitive. The slightest touch of clothing or even a change in temperature can produce a flare of pain.

Postherpetic neuralgia affects half of people older than age 60 who get shingles and 75 percent of people older than age 70 with shingles. For many people, the condition gradually disappears on its own, but this can take several years.

Unknown causes

Sometimes, chronic pain develops for no apparent reason. Despite repeated tests, your doctor isn't able to link it to an identifiable physical cause or condition. This doesn't mean that the pain doesn't exist. It simply means that your pain may be associated with factors that are difficult to diagnose.

Your health also is affected by the interaction of your mind and body. Among some people, psychological issues can play a major role in chronic pain. For example, people who've endured sexual abuse or other kinds of physical abuse appear to have a greater risk for development of chronic pelvic or abdominal pain. It's unknown whether the pain is the result of physical injuries or if it stems from emotional scars or stress. It may be due to a combination of factors.

Is cancer pain chronic?

Many people view cancer pain as a form of chronic pain, but it's not. Cancer pain is generally considered an acute form of pain because it's caused by tissue damage. The pain often stems from tumors that press against nerves or that interfere with blood flow or the functioning of your internal organs. Or, it may result from treatments aimed at curing the disease.

Because the pain is acute, management for this type of pain is different. However, some of the techniques used to control chronic pain also can be beneficial in managing cancer pain.

Chapter 3

Cycles of Chronic Pain

*P*eople living with chronic pain often compare their lives to a roller coaster ride. There are good days when you feel uplifted and in control, followed by bad days when your mood sinks and you feel helpless. Rarely does pain stay at an even level. It fluctuates. Pain also doesn't have any boundaries. When a part of you is in pain, your whole body reacts.

As you try to understand, accept and manage your condition, your behavior and emotions may go through a series of ups and downs. This is especially true if you have debilitating pain. Often, these behavioral and emotional changes follow a predictable pattern.

Behavioral cycle

One of the first noticeable effects of chronic pain is the change it brings in your day-to-day activities. Regular tasks often become more difficult, even impossible.

The following scenario is an example of how chronic pain often works—how it can easily alter your routine and behavior.

Stage 1: Decrease in activity
Because of your pain, just getting the yard rake down from the garage attic—much less raking the entire yard—seems like too big a chore.

So instead, you let the leaves fall. But every time you pass by a window, you're reminded of what you can't do.

You could hire someone to rake the yard, but that would cost money. You could have your family do it, but they might feel resentful that you're not out helping them. Plus, you don't like the idea of watching others take over your responsibilities.

So, you wait for a day when you feel better.

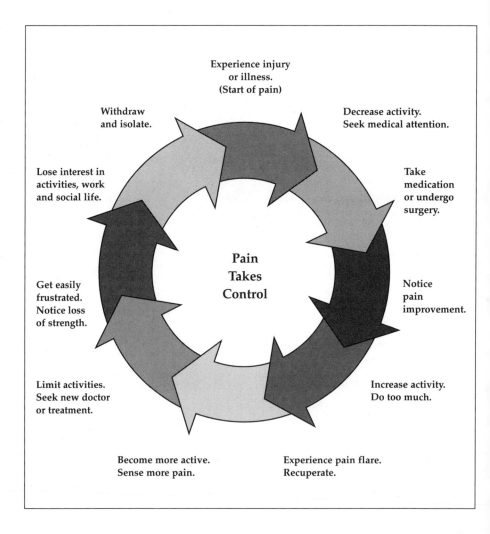

Uncontrolled chronic pain commonly causes this pattern of behavior, beginning at the top of the circle and moving clockwise.

Stage 2: Increase in activity

When the day arrives when your pain seems to be improving, you rake the yard. But you also run errands, clean the garage and go out to dinner with friends.

You put in a day best fit for a superhero. But as long as you're feeling well, why not catch up on all those things you've been neglecting?

Stage 3: More pain, less activity

The next day, you can hardly move. You feel worse than you did before your superheroic day. You chastise yourself for trying to do too much at one time and spend the next few days resting and trying to recuperate.

Eventually, you begin to feel better. But as you start to become more active, your pain worsens. Thinking that the only way to control your pain is to limit all physical activity, you turn over many of your daily chores to family members or friends and spend more time in bed or on the couch.

Meanwhile, the leaves continue to fall, friends keep calling and you don't feel up to doing anything.

Stage 4: Loss of strength and physical deconditioning

The time you spend lying around is making you tired, weak and less able to finish up those leaves. Because of your long stretch of inactivity, your stamina is leaving you. You get fatigued easily. Even the thought of physical labor is daunting.

Stage 5: Withdrawal and isolation

You find yourself spending more time alone and less time with those who care about you. Because you've stopped going out with your friends, they've stopped calling. They figure that you'd just turn them down anyway, so why bother?

Your family has become accustomed to doing things without you. Not only can they now rake the yard without your help but also they've started going out to dinner or attending social events without you. They think they're accommodating you by not "forcing" you to go.

You retreat even further from your family, friends and favorite activities. Eventually, a day comes when you begin to feel a little better. It's followed by another good day, and you feel optimistic that your condition may finally be improving. But once again, your pain flares, and the cycle repeats itself.

Communicating your pain

When you're in pain, others can often tell it by your actions. These actions, called pain behaviors, refer to the things you do or say to signal people that you're experiencing pain. They're a way of calling attention to your pain—either consciously or unconsciously.

Pain behaviors are a natural response to pain. During an initial period of acute pain, they may help reduce your pain. But over time they become ineffective. For people with chronic pain, pain behaviors often become a habit.

Common pain behaviors include:
• Limping
• Crying
• Groaning
• Grimacing
• Limiting activity
• Staying in bed
• Using protective posture
• Talking about pain or surgery
• Withdrawing from others

People around you generally react in one of two ways to pain behaviors: They become annoyed by them—"Not this again"—or they become overly attentive to the behaviors—"Here, let me do that." Either response creates an unequal relationship in which people tend to focus more on your behaviors than on your thoughts or feelings.

Pain behaviors also consume a lot of energy that could be channeled into other, more productive ventures, such as taking steps to manage your pain.

The bottom line is that pain behaviors don't help your situation and they can harm your personal relationships as well as your self-esteem.

Emotional cycle

Just as your behavior fluctuates when you're in pain, so do your emotions. Often, the two go hand in hand—the more you're able to do, the better your mood, and the less you're able to do, the worse your mood. Like your behaviors, your emotions also tend to follow a cyclic pattern.

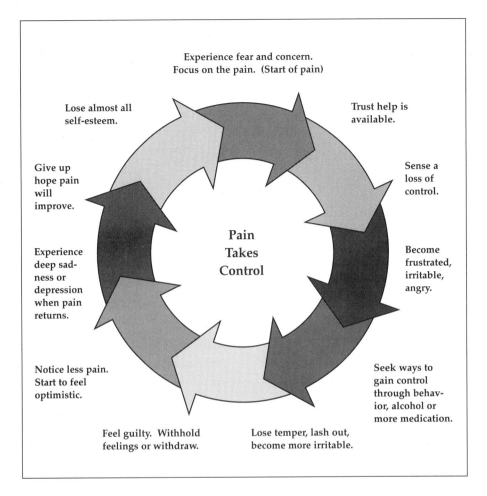

Uncontrolled chronic pain commonly causes this pattern of emotions, beginning at the top of the circle and moving clockwise.

Stage 1: Fear and concern

When you first experience your pain, you're fearful and concerned. You worry that your pain may be a symptom of a disabling or serious disease. Your pain becomes the focus of your attention. The more you worry about it, the worse it seems to get, and in turn, the harder it becomes to ignore.

Stage 2: Hope and promise

When you finally learn what's triggering your pain, your fear and concern are replaced with hope that your doctor will be able to make the pain disappear and your life will soon return to normal. If your doctor isn't able to find a cause, at least knowing that your pain isn't a symptom of a life-threatening condition makes you feel better.

You think that curing your pain is a reasonable request. In today's society, when something breaks you expect someone to fix it. But repairing your body is far more complicated than fixing your car or a household appliance. When the pain continues to linger despite repeated trips to various doctors, your hope starts to diminish.

Stage 3: Anger and frustration

You become dejected and depressed over the state of your life. This is the stage when you ask, "Why me?" and "What did I do to deserve this?" On some level, you may know that the pain isn't a punishment. But, still, you feel as if you've done something wrong and now you're paying the consequences.

You also may find it easy to vent your frustration on others—your doctors, your insurance representatives and even your own family and friends. But it's displaced anger. What's upsetting you may be the long waits at your doctor's office, the bill at the end of each visit, increased dependence on others, a sense of loss of control or, perhaps most of all, no relief from your pain.

As your life feels less and less your own, you may seek to gain control in other, destructive ways, such as increasing your pain medication or using alcohol. You may become more irritable with the people who are trying their best to help you.

Stage 4: Guilt and withdrawal

You feel guilty over the things you've said and done. Instead of communicating this guilt, you withdraw from people so you won't take your anger out on them.

You also feel guilty because you aren't able to do your full share anymore. Your spouse or children have taken over some of your duties, such as parenting responsibilities, cleaning the house or raking the yard. At work, you can't keep up your normal pace and your coworkers are having to lend you a hand. Instead of venting your frustrations, you may start to withhold your emotions and keep them bottled up inside.

Stage 5: Renewed hope, followed by depression

Gradually, or perhaps rather suddenly, you feel better. You're optimistic

Overachiever's curse

Living with chronic pain isn't easy for anyone. But it can be especially difficult if you've prided yourself on being a perfectionist or always on the go.

If you're the sort of person who gets things done and is always called on to complete a project on time, make the cookies for the bake sale or coach the Little League team, being unable to do your part because of your pain can be devastating.

When chronic pain hits, an overachiever often has to settle for being just like everyone else. This causes some people to fall victim to "all-or-nothing" thinking. If they can't head the committee, they don't even want to be involved. They completely dismiss themselves from their normal activities and become very withdrawn and depressed.

that your condition is finally improving or the new treatment you're trying is working. Excitedly, you start getting back into your old routine. But after a time, the pain returns and you become deeply disappointed and lose all hope of recovery. You feel depressed and find that you can hardly make it out of bed in the morning. Things that used to matter to you, such as your appearance or attending family or social activities, don't seem important.

You begin to feel as though you're no longer loved or needed, and your self-esteem hits an all-time low. You may even begin to wonder if you're deserving of love and attention. As you draw deeper inside yourself, your pain becomes the focus of all of your attention. Fear, isolation and depression, coupled with days with nothing to do, make the pain feel even worse. The severity of your pain finally forces you to look for other forms of treatment, setting you up for a repeat of the cycle.

Your family's responses

Your pain, and how you react to it, also affects your family. Their responses to your behavior and emotions can take on parallel cycles of their own.

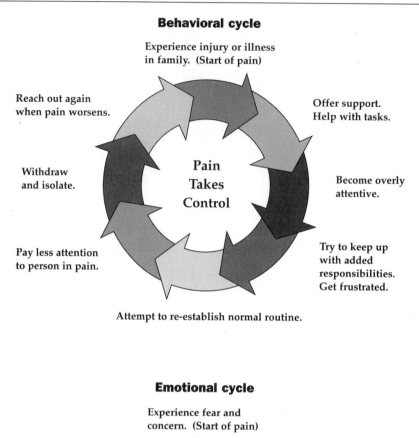

Behavioral cycle

Experience injury or illness
in family. (Start of pain)

Reach out again
when pain worsens.

Offer support.
Help with tasks.

Withdraw
and isolate.

**Pain
Takes
Control**

Become overly
attentive.

Pay less attention
to person in pain.

Try to keep up
with added
responsibilities.
Get frustrated.

Attempt to re-establish normal routine.

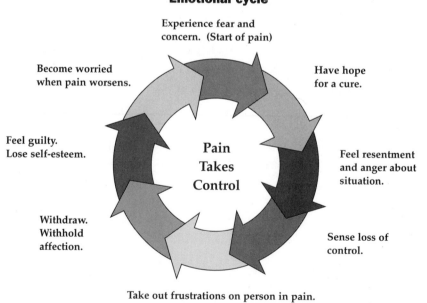

Emotional cycle

Experience fear and
concern. (Start of pain)

Become worried
when pain worsens.

Have hope
for a cure.

Feel guilty.
Lose self-esteem.

**Pain
Takes
Control**

Feel resentment
and anger about
situation.

Withdraw.
Withhold
affection.

Sense loss of
control.

Take out frustrations on person in pain.

**Family members commonly experience patterns of behavior and emotion that are similar to those
of the person in pain.**

Family behaviors

When chronic pain first becomes a problem, family members generally show a great deal of support. They're often increasingly attentive to you, making sure you're as comfortable as possible. They do more tasks around the house so you can relax and "get better."

Family members also become vigilant in assessing your pain and keeping track of the activities that seem to make it better or worse. They observe and monitor you closely, in an attempt to help lessen your pain and help your doctor make a diagnosis.

When your pain doesn't improve, your family's patience may start to wear thin. At this stage, they begin to resent the extra burden they've been handed. And though most family members realize that it's not your fault, it becomes difficult to separate the person from the pain. They may begin to withdraw themselves and pay less attention to you.

Family emotions

Family members often go through the very same emotions you do. Initially, they fear the cause of your pain. Later, when your treatment doesn't seem to be working and they're shouldering more responsibilities, they become angry and begin to ask, "Why me?"—or more appropriately—"Why us?"

Just as you do, family members often feel a loss of control over their daily lives and normal routine. This frustration can lead them to withhold affection because they're angry at the situation facing them. They may unintentionally take this anger out on you.

They feel bad about being angry with you and, in turn, start to feel bad about themselves and how they're acting. "I'm not a good person" and "I should be able to handle this" are common thoughts. Their guilt often leads to increased attentiveness and care, beginning the behavioral cycle again.

Unfortunately, even though you and your family share common feelings, you may find these feelings difficult to talk about. Your family members fear it will sound like they're blaming you for your pain. They also don't want to come across as being selfish and inconsiderate. You have many of the same fears. The silence, however, often brings more resentment and frustration.

Breaking the cycles

You may think that the cycles of chronic pain will never end. But you can break free of them. The downward spiral that often accompanies chronic pain occurs when all of your attention is focused on your pain. To accommodate your pain, you change your life, often in ways you don't like.

By learning how to manage your pain so it's no longer the focus of your attention, you can concentrate on the things that give you pleasure and satisfaction. This renewed feeling of control over your life will help you end the pain cycles.

Chapter 4

Recognizing the Costs
of Chronic Pain

Not everyone experiences the rippling effects of chronic pain.
Some people can live with their pain without it taking a toll on
their daily lives and overall health. Others aren't as lucky. If
you're suffering significantly because of your pain, you're not alone.

This chapter details the personal and economic costs associated with
chronic pain. It's not an upbeat discussion. But the good news is that
the story doesn't end here. This book is about improving your quality
of life, despite your pain. In the chapters that follow, you'll learn what
you can do to help minimize these personal and economic costs and, in
some cases, avoid them.

Physical deconditioning

You know that you need regular physical activity to stay healthy. But
when you're in pain, you don't feel like being active. Like many people,
you may have started an exercise routine. But you did too much the
first day. The next day you felt so much worse that the thought of exercising again was more than you could handle.

Risks of inactivity include:

Unhealthy body composition. Inactivity can lead to increased body
fat. In addition to weight gain, a higher proportion of body fat increases
your risk of cardiovascular disease and diabetes. Because many physical

activities, such as walking, are weight-bearing, inactivity also can weaken your bones and lead to a higher risk of osteoporosis.

Weakened immune system. This can increase your susceptibility to infections, such as colds and flu.

As your body becomes more deconditioned, you begin to feel as though you may never be healthy again.

Loss of sleep

Chronic pain reduces restful sleep. According to a Gallup poll sponsored by the National Sleep Foundation, 62 percent of people with chronic pain reported awaking too early because of their pain and being unable to fall back to sleep.

In addition to the direct effect of pain on sleep, other factors associated with chronic pain can indirectly influence how much and how well you rest:

Lack of physical activity. Inactivity makes it more difficult for you to relax and sleep well.

Excessive alcohol. Drinking too much alcohol reduces restorative sleep by interfering with your brain's ability to produce adequate periods of deep sleep.

Medications. Some pain medications can stimulate your nervous system so you don't feel tired.

When you don't get adequate sleep, you lack energy, are more easily irritated and aren't able to cope as well with pain and stress. Regular or extended bouts of sleeplessness also can wear on your health. Your body needs restorative sleep to keep all of its systems working properly.

Emotional upheaval

Pain can play havoc on your emotions. One minute you may feel fine, the next your world may feel as though it's been torn apart. For some people, that's a literal account. An accident or fall can change your life in an instant. For others, the development of chronic pain is a more gradual process. In either case, the pain has divided your life into two distinct parts—life as you knew it before the pain and life as you now know it afterward.

In your new life, you may feel powerless and trapped. Your emotions may range from fear and frustration to anger and apathy. Dealing with these emotions is often difficult. You long for your life before the pain, but the more you do so, the more frustrated or angry you become.

When you're in pain, your sense of security also disappears. What if I lose my job? Will my family understand? How do my friends think about me? The more anxious you become about your situation, the more stressed you feel.

Over time, stress can take its toll, increasing your risk for headaches, intestinal disorders and cardiovascular problems, including a form of chest pain (angina) and an increased heart rate.

Depression

Depression and chronic pain often go hand in hand. Emotional strain, combined with persistent pain, creates a sinkhole that can be difficult to escape. Studies indicate that up to half of people with chronic pain experience mild to severe depression.

It's natural to experience some symptoms of depression when chronic pain first develops or for short periods afterward. Your pain itself also may cause symptoms associated with depression, such as slowed movements or loss of energy. But if your symptoms linger for several months or they become severe, you may be experiencing depression.

A person with depression may have some, most or all of these symptoms:
- Lasting sadness
- Loss of interest or pleasure in most activities
- Neglect of personal responsibilities and personal care
- Irritability and mood swings
- Change in appetite and weight gain or loss
- Recurrent morning awakening or other changes in sleep patterns
- Feelings of restlessness
- Feelings of hopelessness or helplessness
- Extreme fatigue, loss of energy or slowed movements
- Continual negative view of the world and others
- Feelings of worthlessness or inappropriate feelings of guilt
- Decreased concentration, attention and memory
- Decreased sex drive

- Increased focus on physical complaints
- Thoughts of death or suicide

It's unknown what causes most depression, but psychological and biological factors may play a role. Genetic factors, imbalances in certain body or brain chemicals or abnormal sleep behaviors also may give rise to depression.

Regardless of the cause, depression is a complex condition that can make your pain feel worse. That's because it's difficult to separate your mood from your pain intensity. People who are depressed often report stronger, longer lasting and more severe pain than people who aren't depressed.

Depression should be treated. With treatment, up to 80 percent of people with depression show improvement, usually in a matter of weeks. However, many people don't receive treatment because they're unaware of their condition or they don't view depression as an illness. Instead, they think that they can handle the condition on their own.

Difficulties at work

At first, your employer may have been sympathetic to your pain. Perhaps your boss made your workload lighter to accommodate you, or your coworkers pitched in to help you out. But, often, as the pain progresses, things change.

Troubles with a boss or lack of understanding from coworkers can make work a stressful place. This only adds to the pain. If you're having trouble keeping up, you also may fear that you'll lose your job.

Often, the result is some difficult decisions. Options to control your pain and stress may include requesting a shorter workday or changing jobs. But that may not be possible or may involve some unacceptable compromises. For example, another, less stressful position may not offer a comparable salary or insurance benefits.

Financial strain

Medical bills, medications and lost days of work can strain your finances. If your pain has forced you to quit your job, your current income may not be sufficient to meet your expenses. To make up for the drop in income, perhaps your spouse has found a new job or is working additional hours.

Some people reach a point where they need to see a financial consultant or move to a less expensive home to avoid bankruptcy. All of these financial worries can compound your pain and further drain your sense of self-esteem.

Damaged relationships

People who were once supportive and always offering to lend a hand may not be around as much. They've gone on with their lives and seem to have less time for you.

Family relationships also seem strained. Even though your family knows you're not to blame, they're frustrated for the way your pain has changed your life and theirs.

Communication in general is difficult. You get easily irritated and find yourself taking out your emotions on those closest to you. Or, to the contrary, you withdraw and don't share your thoughts or feelings at all.

Your pain also may be straining your sexual relationship. Some people experience sexual difficulties, due to pain, stress or medications. Others avoid intimacy and sexual intercourse because they no longer feel sexually attractive or they fear intercourse will increase their pain.

Chemical dependency

Reliance on medications can be a troublesome side effect of chronic pain. Signs and symptoms that medication use may be a problem include:
- A preoccupation with taking medications
- Taking more medication than prescribed
- Use of more than one physician or pharmacy to get medication
- Hiding medications or being secretive about their use
- Using someone else's medication
- Forgetting when you last took a pill
- Use of an emergency room to get medication
- Drowsiness or periods when you can't recall events

Some people also turn to alcohol or illicit drugs to find relief from their pain and pressures. These drugs can lead to chemical dependency as well. Plus, when you combine prescription medications with other drugs, including alcohol, you increase your risk for dangerous side effects.

Types of dependency

There are three forms of chemical dependency:

Increased tolerance. As your body becomes accustomed to a drug, it can lose its effectiveness. To receive the same degree of relief, you start taking more of the drug than recommended.

Physical dependence. You experience physical withdrawal symptoms when use of the drug is abruptly stopped or its dosage substantially reduced. To control your pain, you rely on your medication at regular intervals.

Addiction. Addiction involves both physical and psychological dependence on a drug. This is possible with prescription medications as well as alcohol and illicit drugs, such as marijuana or cocaine. You become fixated or obsessed with a drug, leading to loss of control over its use.

Side effects of dependency

Serious problems can develop when drugs are misused:

Impaired mental functioning. This includes drowsiness, an inability to concentrate and loss of memory.

Physical complications. Damage may occur to many of your organs, including your heart, blood vessels, liver, kidneys and brain.

Emotional distress. You may regularly experience feelings of anxiety, irritability, apathy and depression.

Taking one step at a time

Overcoming the costs of your pain may seem daunting. But remember that the problems and conditions that chronic pain can produce are often linked. And even a few small steps can bring noticeable results. For example, making an effort to reduce daily stress can have a positive effect on your physical health, sleep, work, personal relationships, finances and depression. As you begin to see improvements, the task ahead may seem more obtainable.

Chapter 5

Taking Control
of Your Pain

T here are many people with chronic pain enjoying active and productive lives. If you aren't among them, there's no reason you can't be. But it's up to you to make it happen.

There aren't any quick fixes for chronic pain. And often, there's only so much doctors can do. *You* are the key ingredient. If you want your life to improve, you need to lead the way.

You may not like the fact that you have chronic pain. No one does. But clinging to unrealistic hopes or expectations will only prolong your frustration and contribute to your feelings of helplessness.

Understanding your role

The first and most important step in controlling your pain is accepting the fact that you may always have pain. Some people are able to significantly reduce or eliminate their pain. But for most people with chronic pain, their pain will always be a part of their life.

Managing chronic pain isn't about making your pain disappear. It's about learning how to keep your pain at a tolerable level. It's about enjoying life again, despite your pain. And it's about accepting that only you can control your future.

The choice is yours to make. You can continue to put up with your pain or you can do something about it. You can dwell on your discomfort or you can look for solutions.

This can be frightening. For months or even years you may have pinned your hopes on others to treat your condition or tell you what to do. But just as you've learned how to manage other things in your life—your finances, your job or your family—you can learn to manage your pain.

The remainder of this book focuses on specific lifestyle issues and pain management therapies that can help you better understand and control your pain. Each small step you take in your new role as pain manager will boost your self-confidence and strengthen your faith in your abilities.

Finding the right doctor

Being in charge of your pain doesn't mean that you can't or shouldn't seek help from others. Having people around who can help you when you have questions or need assistance is important. A doctor can be especially helpful. But make sure it's a doctor who understands your condition and believes in what you're doing.

The right doctor for you could be your family physician or a specialist who's overseeing your condition. Or, you may want to see a physician or a psychologist who specializes in pain management. If you're not sure where to find a pain specialist, ask your doctor to refer you to one.

Before selecting a new doctor, however, check with your health insurance provider to make sure the physician is covered under your policy.

When selecting a doctor, look for someone with these characteristics:
• Is knowledgeable about chronic pain
• Wants to help
• Listens well
• Makes you feel at ease
• Encourages you to ask questions
• Seems honest and trustworthy
• Allows you to disagree
• Is willing to talk with family or friends

In addition to finding the right doctor, make an effort to learn all that you can about your condition and your pain. This will make it easier for the two of you to work together as a team (see "Where to get more information").

Where to get more information

There are many places you can go to learn more about chronic pain or your specific medical condition. Reference areas at most libraries include medical dictionaries, books on health topics and health magazines. You also can browse through the health section in your local bookstore.

If you have a personal computer and access to the Internet, many medical centers, government agencies, nonprofit health organizations and publishers use the World Wide Web as a fast and easy way to provide in-depth health information.

But be cautious about what you read or purchase. Just because something has been published or it's on the Internet isn't a guarantee that the information is accurate or reliable. Anyone who has the necessary hardware and software can publish a Web page or offer medical advice. And the Internet has a way of making all health information appear equal.

Look for reliable sources for your health information. Is it from a respected publication or organization? Has it been reviewed by health professionals? Is it current?

To help you get started, in the back of the book is a list of specific organizations you can call, write or access via your computer for more information on chronic pain (see "Additional Resources," page 167).

A Note of Caution: It's important to be informed about your health. However, spending too much time reading about your condition or discussing your pain can be counterproductive. It constantly draws your attention to your pain, instead of away from it.

Keeping a journal

As you learn techniques to manage your pain, you should see an increase in your activity level and, perhaps, a decrease in your pain level. A daily journal helps you track your progress and determine the therapies or activities that seem to be helping you the most. A journal also is an easy way to keep track of goals you want to achieve and your progress in reaching them.

Many people think that their pain isn't influenced by factors such as work, stress, sleep or physical activity. But after a few months of tracking their pain levels and their activities, they begin to notice some common patterns.

In addition, a journal can be a great way to express your feelings about your pain or other things that are happening in your life. Writing your thoughts and feelings on paper helps you organize and sort through problems and emotions and get them "off your chest," similar to the way you feel after a good heart-to-heart visit with a friend or family member.

Your journal can be as simple or as detailed as you like (see "Whatever works," page 46). However, try to include the following information, especially when you first begin. As you gain a better understanding of your pain and learn how to manage it, you may find it more helpful to focus on just one or two areas.

Pain level and activities

Health care professionals typically measure pain on a scale of 0 to 10, with 0 being no pain and 10 being the worst imaginable pain (see "Rating your pain"). Using this scale as your guide, a couple of times a day rate your pain level and record it in your journal. In addition, briefly state your activities that day and when you did them.

You can do this whenever it's convenient, but keep the times consistent. Many people choose to record their pain level in the morning when they wake up, after lunch and in the evening before bed.

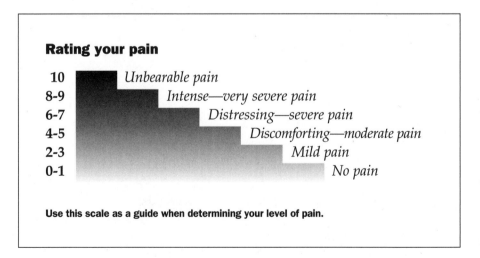

Rating your pain

10	Unbearable pain
8-9	Intense—very severe pain
6-7	Distressing—severe pain
4-5	Discomforting—moderate pain
2-3	Mild pain
0-1	No pain

Use this scale as a guide when determining your level of pain.

Keeping a log of your pain levels and activities allows you to:

Learn your pain pattern. Most people find that the changes in their pain levels are quite consistent. For example, your pain may generally be at its lowest level in the morning and its highest level in the evening. Recording your pain levels helps you determine your pain pattern.

Link your pain with your activities. If your pain is always the worst in the evening, why? Look to see if certain activities seem to correlate with an increase or a decrease in your pain level. Are you sitting or standing too long? Is your rush to get dinner ready a contributing factor? Or are you just tired?

Identify flares. Recording your pain levels helps draw attention to inconsistencies. If your pain level at noon is normally a 3 and one day it's a 6, seeing the difference may prompt you to think about your morning. Did you do something different? Did you have an especially stressful morning?

See your progress. If you feel you aren't making progress, reading your journal may help you to realize that your life has improved, even though the process may seem slow. Your journal also may give you clues as to why some areas remain difficult for you.

Mood

On a scale of 0 to 10, with 0 being poor and 10 being excellent, rate your mood. This exercise helps you realize that even though your pain and your mood are closely aligned, they aren't bound together.

Typically, the worse your pain, the worse your mood, and vice versa. However, as you begin to feel more in control of your pain you may find your mood improving at a faster rate than the improvement in your pain levels. Rating your mood helps you realize that even though you may not be able to eliminate your pain, you can learn to live with it and still be happy.

Sleep

A good night's sleep better equips you to handle your day. However, getting enough sleep can be difficult because your pain may keep you up at night. In contrast, some people spend too much time in bed. This also can reduce your pain tolerance.

Once a day, record how many hours you slept during the past 24 hours. Eight hours is average, but the amount of sleep each person needs varies. Your goal should be to feel rested when you awake.

In Chapter 11 (page 101), we talk more about the importance of sleep and give you tips to help you sleep better.

Whatever works

There is no right or wrong when it comes to keeping a journal. Some people like to simply jot down their thoughts, others prefer a worksheet format. This is just one example of how your journal might look and the information to include.

Date: January 1   Hours slept: 7

	7:00 a.m.	1:00 p.m.	10:00 p.m.
Pain level	5	4	6
Mood	7	6	4

Morning
5:00-5:30 Coffee and breakfast
5:30-7:00 Exercised and got ready for work
7:30-11:00 Work
11:30-12:30 15-minute walk and lunch

Afternoon and evening
12:30-4:30 Work
5:00-5:30 Read paper and
    went through mail
5:30-6:00 Relaxation exercises
6:00-7:00 Dinner
7:00-8:30 Did errands and
    attended meeting
9:00-10:00 Wrote in journal
    and got ready for bed.

Comments/thoughts: I slept a little better last night. I still woke up at 5:00 but I didn't feel so tired. I also seem to have more energy at work. I think the morning exercises are helping. Evenings are still a problem. I know I need to rest more but it seems there are just too many things to do.

Setting SMART goals

When you're in pain, it's easy for the pain to become the center of all of your attention. Other things in life that were important to you, or that you were trying to achieve, may have taken a back seat to the pain.

Setting goals helps divert your attention from your pain and provides an opportunity to think about your lifestyle, and what you can do to better manage your pain. Goals also give you something to strive for.

But goal setting isn't as easy as it may sound. You simply can't identify a couple things you want and expect them to occur. You'll only be setting yourself up for disappointment.

The key is to set goals that are SMART:

Specific. State exactly what you want to achieve, how you're going to do it and when you want to achieve it. To begin with, set goals that you can achieve within a week to a month. It's easy to give up on goals that take too long to reach.

If you have a large goal, break it down into a series of smaller weekly or daily goals. After you achieve one of the smaller goals, move on to the next.

Measurable. A goal doesn't do you any good if there's no way of telling if you've achieved it. "I want to feel better" isn't a good goal. It's not specific and it's difficult to measure. "I want to work 8 hours each day" is a good goal. It's specific and it's measurable.

Attainable. Ask yourself if the goal is within reasonable reach. For instance, completing a marathon may not be an achievable goal if you've never run before. But completing a 3K run may be attainable.

Realistic. Is the goal realistic for you? The purpose of goal setting is to take your focus off your pain and think about your future. But you can't ignore your limitations. Your goals need to be within your capabilities. If you've suffered a serious back injury, a goal of returning to work as a bricklayer may not be realistic. Instead, your goal might be to find a sales or consulting job in a related field. Or, you might consider going back to school and making a new degree your goal.

Trackable. Being able to track your progress encourages you to keep going and reach your goal. Look for ways to chart your improvements.

Here's how

These are examples of goals that follow the SMART formula:

Goal: Eliminate use of over-the-counter pain medications
When I want to achieve it: 2 weeks
How I'm going to do it: Plan my day to include exercise, pace myself at work and take frequent breaks, use relaxation techniques
How I'm going to measure it: Each day, record in my journal the medication I took and how much

Goal: Exercise 40 minutes each day
When I want to achieve it: 4 weeks
How I'm going to do it: Stretch and do strengthening exercises 15 minutes in the morning, walk 10 minutes during my lunch hour, bicycle 15 minutes in the evening
How I'm going to measure it: Record in my journal when I exercised and for how long

Your turn

Think carefully about some short-term or long-term goals you want to achieve. If you have some in mind, you can write them down now. Otherwise, finish reading this book and return to this section when you're done.

As you work on your goals, you may find that the strategies you use to reach one goal will help you with others.

Once you've completed your goals, put them somewhere you can see them. Seeing your goals can help motivate you. As you accomplish your goals, set new ones.

Physical activity

Goal: _____

_____

When I want to achieve it: _____

_____

How I'm going to do it: _____

_____

How I'm going to measure it: _____

_____

Goal: _____

_____

When I want to achieve it: _____

_____

How I'm going to do it: _____

_____

How I'm going to measure it: _____

_____

Emotions and behavior

Goal: _____

_____

When I want to achieve it: _____

_____

How I'm going to do it: _____

_____

How I'm going to measure it: _____

_____

Goal: _____

_____

When I want to achieve it: _____

_____

How I'm going to do it: _____

_____

How I'm going to measure it: _____

_____

Stress and relaxation

Goal: _____

_____

When I want to achieve it: _____

_____

How I'm going to do it: _____

_____

How I'm going to measure it: _____

_____

Goal: _____

_____

When I want to achieve it: _____

_____

How I'm going to do it: _____

_____

How I'm going to measure it: _____

_____

Family and friends
Goal: _____

_____

When I want to achieve it: _____

_____

How I'm going to do it: _____

_____

How I'm going to measure it: _____

_____

Goal: _____

_____

When I want to achieve it: _____

_____

How I'm going to do it: _____

_____

How I'm going to measure it: _____

_____

Leisure and recreation
Goal: _____

_____

When I want to achieve it: _____

_____

How I'm going to do it: _____

_____

How I'm going to measure it: _____

_____

Goal: _____

_____

When I want to achieve it: _____

_____

How I'm going to do it: _____

_____

How I'm going to measure it: _____

_____

Work

Goal: _____

_____

When I want to achieve it: _____

_____

How I'm going to do it: _____

_____

How I'm going to measure it: _____

_____

Goal: _____

_____

When I want to achieve it: _____

_____

How I'm going to do it: _____

_____

How I'm going to measure it: _____

_____

Medication

Goal: _____

_____

When I want to achieve it: _____

_____

How I'm going to do it: _____

_____

How I'm going to measure it: _____

_____

Goal: _____

_____

When I want to achieve it: _____

_____

How I'm going to do it: _____

_____

How I'm going to measure it: _____

_____

You may be surprised

Some people are resistant to keeping a journal or setting goals. They feel it sounds like too much work or it'll take up too much time. Or, they think it sounds "silly." If you happen to be one of these people, ask yourself a couple of questions. Is your present strategy—the things you're doing now to manage your pain—working? Is there any harm that can result from trying these new techniques?

Many people who are resistant to keeping a journal or goal setting, or are skeptical of their benefits, eventually find the processes helpful.

Chapter 6

Getting Moving With Exercise

*T*here was a time when people with chronic pain were told to avoid physical activity for fear it would damage their joints and muscles and worsen their pain. No more.

When you aren't active, you begin to lose muscle tone and strength and your cardiovascular system works less efficiently. Inactivity also increases your risk for high blood pressure, high cholesterol and diabetes, putting you at increased risk for heart attack and stroke. In addition, inactivity can disrupt your sleep and worsen fatigue, stress and anxiety— as well as your pain.

A common misconception is that exercise increases pain. Just the opposite, exercise can help reduce it. During physical activity, your body releases certain chemicals (endorphins and enkephalins) that block pain signals from reaching your brain. These chemicals also help alleviate anxiety and depression, conditions that can make your pain more difficult to control.

A regular exercise program that includes flexibility, aerobic and strengthening exercises can help improve your fitness and control your pain. Regular exercise also:
- Gives you energy and improves sleep
- Promotes weight loss, reducing stress on your joints
- Increases bone mass, reducing your risk for injury

To help you get and stay active, here's a total fitness program that's safe for almost anyone. To benefit from the program, try to exercise most, if not all, days each week.

Before you get started

It's always a good idea to talk with your doctor before starting any type of physical activity program. If you have another health problem or you're at risk for cardiovascular disease, you may need to take some precautions while you exercise.

It's especially important that you see your doctor if you:
- Have a blood pressure of 160/100 mm Hg or higher
- Have diabetes or heart, lung or kidney disease
- Are a man age 40 years or older or a women age 50 or older and haven't had a recent physical examination
- Have a family history of heart-related problems before age 55
- Are unsure of your health status
- Have previously experienced chest discomfort, shortness of breath or dizziness during exercise or strenuous activity

---

Improving flexibility

Flexibility exercises include simple range-of-motion and stretching exercises. These exercises ease movement in your joints, allowing you to move and carry out daily activities more comfortably. They also prevent your muscles from shortening and tightening, which increase your risk for injury.

Range-of-motion exercises
Include some or all of these exercises in your physical activity program. With each exercise, move slowly and easily.

Neck
- Bring your chin toward your chest, then stretch it up toward the ceiling.

- Tilt your ear to your left shoulder, then right shoulder. Avoid raising your shoulder toward your head.
- Turn your face to the left, then right. Keep your neck, shoulders and trunk straight.

Jaw
- Open your mouth as wide as possible. Close.
- Move your jaw to the right, then left.
- Move your jaw forward, then back.

Shoulders
With your arms at your side:
- Roll your shoulders forward in a circular motion. Reverse.
- Bring your arms forward and over your head. Keep your trunk straight.
- Raise your arms to your sides and over your head. Keep your trunk straight.
- Bring your elbows to shoulder height. Pull your elbows backward and feel a stretch in your chest muscles.

Elbows
- Bend and straighten your elbows.
- Keep your arms next to your body, bend your elbows to make a right angle and turn your palms up and down.

Wrists
- Move your hand from side to side as far as possible, bending at the wrists.
- Move your hand up and down as far as possible, bending at the wrists.

Fingers and thumbs
- Bend your fingers to make a fist. Then fully straighten them.
- Bend your fingers at the knuckles, forming a claw. Then straighten them.
- Bend your thumbs across your palms and pull toward your little fingers.
- Touch the tips of your thumbs to the tips of your little fingers. Open your hands wide. Repeat, touching your thumb to each finger.

Hips

- March in place, bringing your knees up high.
- Raise your leg out to the side. Alternate legs.
- Lift your leg straight back. Don't arch your back. Alternate legs.
- Kick your feet up behind you ("butt" kicks).

Trunk

Standing with your hands on your hips:

- Bend your upper body way to the left. Repeat way to the right.
- Twist your upper body to the right. Repeat to the left. Don't turn your pelvis.

Ankles and feet

Standing with your feet about 12 inches apart:

- Rise on the toes of both your feet. Relax to starting position. Rise on the toes of your right foot. Relax. Rise on the toes of both feet. Relax. Rise on the toes of your left foot. Relax.
- Walk on your heels.
- Walk on your toes.
- Walk heel-to-toe, as though you're on a tightrope.

Stretching exercises

Stretching each time you exercise helps keep your muscles limber, reducing tightness in the muscles. Stretch slowly, holding the position for 30 to 60 seconds, and then slowly release. Breathe deeply and slowly while you stretch.

Never bounce, and stretch only until you feel a noticeable pull. Your muscles respond to over-stretching by tightening—the opposite of what you want them to do.

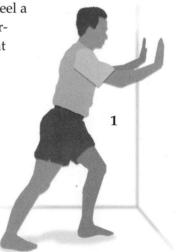

Heel cord stretch (1)

Stand at arm's length from a wall with your palms flat against the wall. Keep one leg back with your knee straight and your heel flat on the floor. Slowly bend your elbows and front knee as you lean toward the wall. Hold and repeat on other leg.

Hamstring stretch (2)

Sit on a low table, or on a chair with your leg propped on another chair in front of you. Without bending your knees, lean forward from your hips. Keep your back straight. Lean forward until you feel a gentle pull in the muscles under your thighs. Hold and repeat on other leg.

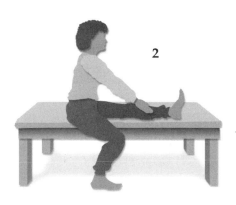

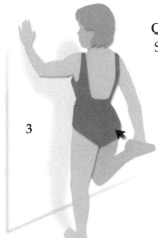

Quadriceps stretch (3)

Stand facing a wall, chair or any support. Place your left hand against the wall or on the support. Grasp the top of your right foot with your right hand and gently pull your thigh back toward your buttocks, until you feel mild tension in the front of your thigh. Hold your abdomen in and keep your back straight. Keep the leg you're stretching directly under you. Relax as you hold the stretch and repeat with other leg.

Hip flexor stretch (4)

Lie on a low table or a bed with your right leg and hip near the edge. Pull your left thigh and knee firmly toward your chest until your lower back flattens against the table or bed. Let your right leg hang in a relaxed position over the edge of the table or bed. Hold and repeat with other leg.

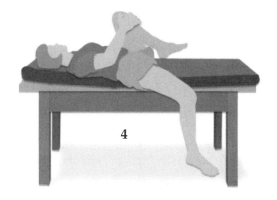

Low back stretch (5)
Lie flat on a firm surface. With your knees
bent, lift one leg at a time toward your
body. Grasp your knees and pull
toward your shoulders. Stop when
you feel a stretch in your lower
back. Hold and return legs,
one at a time, to starting
position. Repeat.

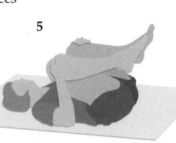

5

Looking for a helping hand?
For help with designing and getting started on your activity
program, contact one of these professionals:

Physical therapist. Most hospitals and clinics have physical
therapists on staff. A physical therapist is trained in the use of
exercise to achieve physical fitness. He or she can help you
select the most appropriate exercises based on the location of
your pain and show you how to do them properly.

Occupational therapist. Occupational therapists also are
available in most hospitals and clinics. An occupational therapist can teach you how to do daily activities in ways that won't
place extra stress on your joints.

Certified exercise therapist. Many health clubs have
employees who are trained in exercise therapy. If you belong to
a health club—or are thinking of joining one—make an appointment to meet with a certified therapist for help with developing
an exercise plan.

Increasing aerobic capacity

Aerobic exercises place added demands on your heart, lungs and muscles,
increasing your heart rate, blood pressure and need for oxygen. These
exercises help your body work more efficiently and reduce your risk for
cardiovascular disease, including heart attack, high blood pressure and
high cholesterol.

Aerobic activity also increases your stamina so you don't become as easily fatigued and you have more energy for daily activities.

Aim for 20 to 40 minutes of moderately intense aerobic activity most, if not all, days each week. For the activity to be beneficial, try to exert a moderate amount of effort (see "Perceived Exertion Scale"). If you've been inactive, start out slowly at an easy pace and gradually increase your time and level of exertion.

There are many forms of aerobic activity. Walking is the most common because it's easy, convenient and cheap. All you need is a good pair of walking shoes.

Other aerobic exercises include:

- Bicycling
- Golfing (walking, not riding)
- Volleyball
- Hiking
- Skiing
- Tennis
- Basketball
- Dancing
- Aerobic dance
- Jogging
- Running
- Swimming and water aerobics

Water aerobics have become increasingly popular among people with chronic pain because water's buoyancy reduces stress on your joints. Water also provides resistance to increase the benefits of aerobic activity. In addition, many people find warm water to be relaxing and soothing to sore muscles and joints.

A disadvantage of water exercises is that they aren't weight–bearing. To maintain bone mass and protect against osteoporosis, combine water exercises with activities such as walking or lifting weights.

Perceived Exertion Scale		
Perceived exertion refers to the total amount of effort, physical stress and fatigue you experience during a physical activity. For the activity to be beneficial to your health, you need to exert a "moderate" to "somewhat strong" effort. That equates to a 3 or 4 on the Perceived Exertion Scale.	0	Nothing at all
	1	Very weak
	2	Weak
	3	Moderate
	4	Somewhat strong
	5	Strong
	6	
	7	Very strong
	8	
	9	
	10	Very, very strong

Building strength

Strong muscles improve your physical fitness and reduce fatigue. They also make it easier to carry out more vigorous types of daily activities, such as carrying laundry up and down the stairs or lifting items at work.

To build muscle, include some or all of these exercises most, if not all, days you exercise. If you're out of shape, begin with 5 repetitions of each and try to build to 25 repetitions.

Abdominal exercises

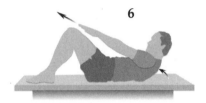
6

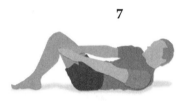
7

Lie on the floor or on a table, with your knees bent (6). Raise your head and shoulders so your shoulder blades lift off the floor or table. Try to keep your head in a neutral position. Hold. Bring your head and shoulders back down. Repeat, reaching both hands toward your left knee (7). Relax. Repeat, reaching both hands toward your right knee.

What about weight lifting?

Lifting weights is an excellent way to strengthen your muscles. However it's best that you work with a physical therapist or fitness trainer in developing and beginning a weight-lifting program. A therapist or trainer will help you select the appropriate weights for your level of fitness and teach you how to lift them properly to avoid injury to your muscles and joints.

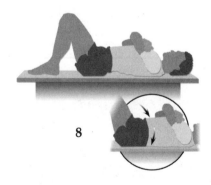
8

Lie on a firm surface with your knees bent (8). Flatten the small of your back against the surface and concentrate on tightening your abdominal muscles. Relax and repeat.

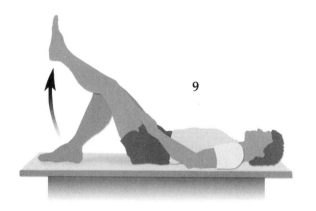

Lie on your back with your right knee bent and your left knee straight (9). Hold your abdominal muscles tight and slowly lower and raise your left leg. Relax and repeat. Reverse legs.

Back exercises

Lie facedown over a large pillow. Position the pillow under your belly button to keep your spine in a neutral position (10). Place your hands behind your hips. Pulling your shoulder blades together, raise your head and chest. Keep your neck relaxed. Return to the starting position and repeat.

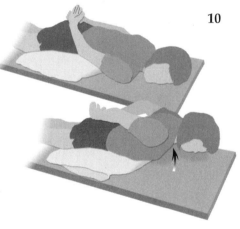

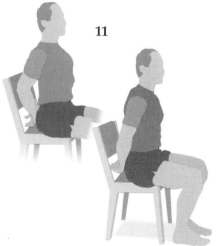

Sit upright in a chair (11). Put your hands on your hips or behind your back and pull your shoulder blades together. Relax and repeat.

Leg exercises

Set up two chairs, one in front of the other (12). Hold on to the back of the chair in front of you and begin to sit in the chair behind you. Partway down, stop and hold your position. Relax and repeat. As you become stronger, try to hold a lower position that is almost, but not quite, seated.

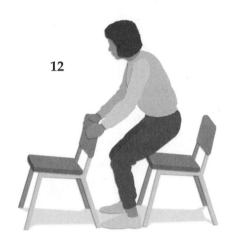

12

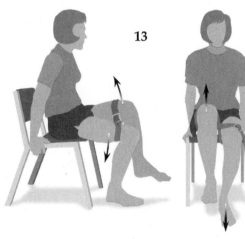

13

Sit on the edge of a chair. Weave a belt around your legs just above your knees so it forms a figure eight (13). Pulling your legs in opposite directions, lift one leg off the floor. Relax. Repeat with other leg.

Sit on the edge of a chair or table. Weave a belt around your ankles so it forms a figure eight (14). Try to straighten one leg while pulling the other foot backward, applying equal force with both legs. Relax. Repeat with other leg.

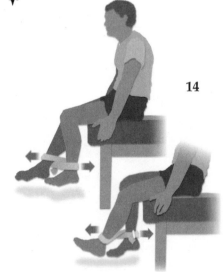

14

Chest and arm exercises

Sit in a sturdy chair that has arms (no wheels), with your feet firmly on the floor. Place your hands on the arms. Push your body up off the surface of the chair using your arms only, not your feet (15). Relax.

15

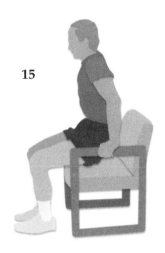

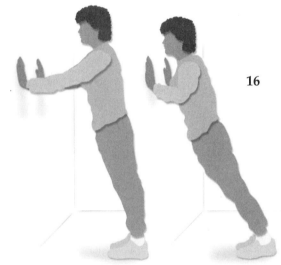

16

Stand facing a wall, far enough away that you can place your palms on the wall with your elbows slightly bent (16). Slowly bend your elbows and lean toward the wall. Straighten your arms and return to a standing position. Repeat. As you build strength, try standing further from the wall.

Perfecting your posture

Good posture places only minimal strain on your joints and muscles. Poor posture, however, can increase stress on some muscles, stretching them or causing them to shorten. When overstretched, your muscles lose their strength. Muscles that are too short are less flexible and more prone to injury and pain.

Avoid poor posture

One extreme of poor posture is the slouch, in which your shoulders are rolled forward. If you perpetually slouch, muscles in your chest shorten, reducing your flexibility.

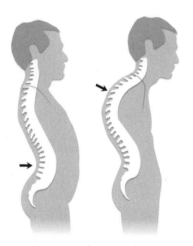

Common forms of poor posture include the slouch posture, right, and swayback posture, left.

The opposite extreme is the swayback. In this position your stomach protrudes too far in front and your buttocks extend too far in the rear. Because of this, your backbone takes on an exaggerated curve between your pelvis and your ribs. Swayback posture puts excessive pressure on your lower back and can contribute to back problems.

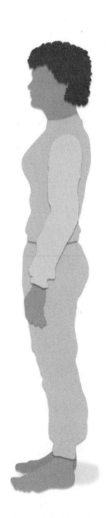

Practice good posture

Good posture will help relax your muscles and may reduce your pain. Throughout the day, including while you exercise, try to maintain good posture.

Good standing posture: Head erect with chin tucked in, chest held high, shoulders relaxed, hips level, knees straight but not locked, feet parallel.

How to straighten up

Here are some tips that can help you improve your posture:

- Sit in a straight-back chair with your back supported.
- Keep your car seat upright so that your hips are at a 90-degree angle.
- Think "tall" when you stand and keep your stomach muscles tight.
- Stand with your weight on both feet.
- Maintain a healthy weight and exercise regularly.
- Sleep on a firm mattress and use a pillow that comfortably supports your neck.
- Wear comfortable shoes without high heels.
- Avoid tight jeans and belts.
- Don't carry bags on your shoulder, such as a purse, that weigh more than 2 pounds.

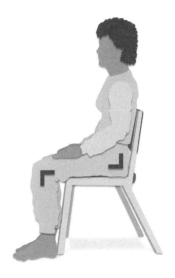

Good sitting posture: Spine and head erect, back and legs at 90-degree angle, natural curves in back maintained.

Keeping your program on track

Regular exercise and good posture can help you stay active and continue to enjoy your favorite leisure activities. As you become more physically fit, you'll also notice an improvement in your energy level. In addition, many people find that as their fitness improves, so does their mood.

To keep up your motivation, do the following:

Set goals

Start with simple goals and then progress to longer-range goals. People who can stay physically active for 6 months usually end up making regular activity a habit. Remember to make your goals realistic and achievable. It's easy to get frustrated and give up on goals that are too ambitious.

Pace yourself

Do a little bit at a time and then rest. When you first exercise you may experience increased discomfort from muscle weakness and joint stiffness. But after a few days, as you gain muscle strength and improve joint flexibility, your pain should start to lessen.

Add variety

Vary what you do to prevent boredom. For example, try alternating walking and bicycling with swimming or a low-impact aerobics dance class. On days when the weather is pleasant, do your flexibility or stretching exercises outside. Consider joining a health club to broaden your access to different forms of physical activity.

Be flexible

If you're traveling or especially busy on a certain day, it's OK to adapt your exercises to accommodate your schedule. If you develop a cold or the flu, take a day or 2 off from your exercise program. Fatigue can increase pain.

Track your progress

Record what you do each time you exercise, how long you do it and how you feel during and after exercising. Recording your efforts helps you work toward your goals as well as remind you that you're making progress.

Reward yourself

Work on developing an internal reward that comes from feelings of accomplishment, self-esteem and control of your own behavior. After each activity session, take 2 to 5 minutes to sit down and relax. Savor the good feelings that exercise gives you, and think about what you've just accomplished. This type of internal reward can help you make a long-term commitment to regular exercise.

External rewards also can help keep you motivated. Upon reaching one of your longer-range goals, you might treat yourself to a new pair of walking shoes or a new cassette tape or CD from one of your favorite musical groups.

Chapter 7

Finding Your Balance

How you organize and go about your day can significantly affect your ability to manage your pain. If you overdo it to meet a deadline at work or overcommit yourself so that you're running from one activity to the next, your body reaches a point where it can't keep up. Fatigue sets in and your pain increases. This can keep you from doing other things that are equally important, such as spending time with family or friends.

The opposite isn't any better—avoiding all activities and spending hours lying around the house. The isolation that this lifestyle produces causes you to focus on only your pain.

The answer is a day that includes a healthful balance—time for work, socializing with family and friends, exercise and recreation, hobbies, relaxation and rest. This can be difficult. Like many people, you may have a lot of constraints on your time. It also isn't easy to change old habits.

Instead of drastically altering your daily routine so it feels uncomfortable, take it one step at a time. Each week, try to incorporate a couple of small changes. Over time, you'll achieve the balance that's right for you.

How does your day balance out?

Think of how you spend a typical weekday. Does it include a balance of activities? The example below shows imbalance. Work consumes most of this person's daytime hours, leaving little time for other activities. The day also doesn't include exercise or time to practice relaxation skills.

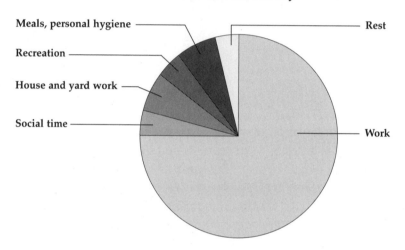

An unbalanced day

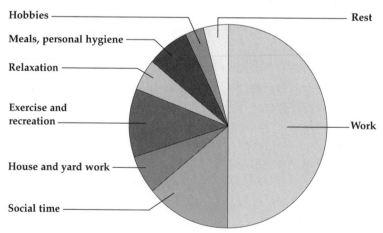

A balanced day

This example shows a balance of daily activities, including time for relaxation and exercise.

During the week and on the weekends, try not to spend a dispropor-tionate amount of time on any one activity, such as more than 8 hours at work. Instead, aim to include as many activities in your day as feels comfortable—including adequate time for rest.

Putting time on your side

For many people, an important step to balancing their day is learning to use time more efficiently. Juggling work, household tasks and social activities can consume large amounts of your day. Procrastination, per-fectionism or overcommitting yourself can make time management even more difficult.

Try these strategies for using your time more wisely:

Plan. Schedule your day so you have time for the things you need to do and those you want to do. Write down all of your activities in a daily planner. Then frequently refer to your planner to make sure you stay on track. At the back of this book (see "Your Personal Planner," page 157) are a week's worth of daily planners to help you get started.

Also, place a central calendar near your telephone to mark down all events and appointments so they don't come as a surprise and to avoid doubling-up on commitments.

Identify. Notice when you "waste" time and avoid these time-wasters. If you can't avoid them, try to make them productive. For example, while waiting for a doctor's appointment or during your daily train commute, listen to a relaxation tape or balance your checkbook.

Prioritize. If you're involved in too many activities that are compet-ing for your time, decide which are the most important and let go of the rest. Your needs come before the wants of others. The consequences of not taking care of yourself likely will be increased pain and fatigue.

Delegate. On days when you have more to do than you can com-fortably handle, seek help from others. Have your son, daughter or spouse do the laundry or prepare dinner.

Evaluate. Think about your day. Are your expectations regarding the number of tasks you can complete in a day realistic?

Educate. Discuss your time needs with those who rely on you the most. If family members, friends or coworkers make unreasonable demands on your time, explain to them that to stay active you need to pace yourself.

Getting more organized

Becoming more organized can save you time so you can incorporate more activities into your day. Organization also helps conserve energy by eliminating wasted steps and unnecessary motions.

Think before you act. Before you begin a task, gather all of the items you need or make a list. For example, keep all of your cleaning supplies in one bucket to avoid multiple trips up and down the stairs. Or list what you need to do before you run errands to avoid a second trip later on.

Keep commonly used items accessible. Organize your work areas at home and at your job so items you use frequently are close at hand. This can save you unnecessary bending or reaching. At home, this might include keeping your spoons and spatulas next to the stove or your wrenches and screwdrivers on a pegboard above your workbench. At work, you might keep your phone adjacent to your computer or frequently used files on your desk.

Reduce clutter. Searching for items takes both time and energy. Organize your counters, cabinets, closets and drawers so you can easily find what you need.

Taking everything in moderation

Moderation involves how much, how long or how fast you do things to avoid "overdoing" or "underdoing" your day. Moderation helps you avoid large swings in your pain level so at the end of each task your pain is near the same level as when you began.

To practice moderation:

Break apart lengthy tasks. Lengthy activities often sap your energy and may increase your pain. Instead of spending all day Saturday planting your garden, spend 1 or 2 hours in the garden over 3 or 4 days. Another example is to divide a 10-hour car trip to visit relatives into 2 days instead of just 1.

Alternate activities. Mix activities that require a lot of effort with those that require only a little energy. After vacuuming one room of the house, sit down and read or pay some bills. Then do a load of laundry. Note times of the day when you have the most energy and the least pain. Plan your priority tasks during these times.

Rest periodically. How often you should take a break depends on the activity. You may find you can do some activities, such as word processing, for 30 minutes to an hour before you need a break. More strenuous tasks, such as mowing the lawn, may require a break every 10 to 20 minutes.

Work at a moderate pace. Instead of rushing to complete a task, take your time and work at a comfortable speed—one in which you feel like you're exerting yourself but not overdoing it. You expend twice as much energy when you work at a fast pace than at a moderate one. It may take you a little longer to get the job done, but in the end you'll feel better.

Changing how you do things

Do you always stand at the kitchen counter while chopping vegetables? Do you balance on your tiptoes and stretch your arm to reach items on high shelves? Do you sit while reading through correspondence at work? If so, do you know why? Chances are, your answer is "That's the way I've always done it."

Adding balance to your day also involves looking for new and more efficient ways to perform everyday tasks, called modification. You want to avoid reaching, bending, twisting or prolonged sitting or standing, actions that consume energy and can aggravate your pain. Instead of standing to cut vegetables, pull up a stool or take the vegetables and cutting board with you and sit at the kitchen table. Instead of stretching to reach an item, use a footstool. Instead of always sitting at your desk, walk around your office while you read.

The less tired you are from doing simple things, the more energy you'll have for more strenuous tasks. Here are examples of some simple ways you can modify your day.

While getting dressed
- Sit down to put on your clothes.
- Place your foot on a chair or stool when tying your shoes.
- Avoid clothes that button or tie in the back.

In the kitchen
- Bend your knees, not your back, to reach items on lower shelves.
- Place one foot on a footstool when standing for long periods, and alternate feet. Whenever possible, sit down.

- Store heavy items within easy reach—between hip and chest level.
- Use electrical appliances when possible, such as an electric can opener, mixer and knife.

Around the house
- Use a long-handled duster for hard-to-reach corners and a long-handled mop to clean your floors.
- Use your legs, not your arm, to move the vacuum.
- Sit on a stool to remove laundry from your dryer.
- Position your bed so you have access to it from three sides. When making your bed, get on your knees to tuck in bed sheets and blankets. Instead of lifting the mattress, push the sheets and blankets between the mattress and box spring.

When outdoors
- Use a wheeled cart to move heavy items.
- Mow your lawn with a self-propelled mower.
- Purchase power tools, such as a power nail driver and screwdriver.
- Use a long-handled rake or hoe to avoid bending.
- Bend your knees when shoveling snow, and use your legs to lift the load. Use a smaller shovel, slide the snow as much as possible and then lift.

Moving your body wisely

Changing how you perform daily activities is based on using your muscles and joints correctly. Proper body mechanics begin with good posture. When you stand or sit, try to keep your shoulders and neck relaxed and your spine aligned properly (see pages 64 and 65).

If you sit for prolonged periods, occasionally elevate your legs by placing your feet on a footstool. Also change positions to shift your weight. This helps divert stress to different muscles.

The same strategies apply to prolonged standing. Shift your weight to change positions and use a low footstool. Place one foot on the stool and frequently alternate your feet. For both sitting and standing, take a 5- to 10-minute break every 30 to 60 minutes.

Here are other examples of proper ways to move:

Reaching

- Avoid excessive arching and twisting of your back.
- Maintain normal spine curves.
- Place one foot forward as close to the object as possible. Grasp the object and pull it slowly to the edge of the shelf by shifting your body weight to your back foot.
- Slowly lower the object to waist level, using your arms. Keep the object as close to you as possible.

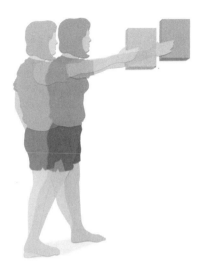

Kneeling

- Keep your feet 8 to 12 inches apart.
- Place one foot forward, and lower your body down to one knee by bending at the hips and knees, keeping your body weight on the balls of your feet.
- If you need, use your arms to help you move in and out of a kneeling position.
- Maintain normal spine curves.
- To progress to full kneeling, lower yourself until both knees are on the floor, and sit back on your heels.
- Reverse the process to stand.

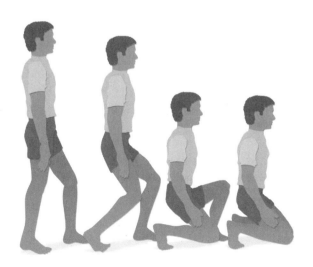

Lifting

- Follow the steps for kneeling, making sure you stand close to the object you're going to lift.
- If the object is heavy, lift it first to your bent knee.
- Lift using your leg muscles to rise from the floor.
- Carry the object close to your body at about waist level. If possible, place your forearms under the object.
- Turn by pivoting your feet. Don't twist at your waist.

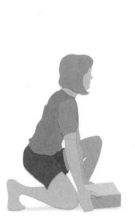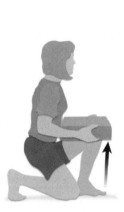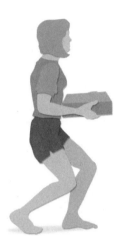

Don't hold your breath

If you've been in an exercise class you may have heard your instructor say, "Don't forget to breathe." And you may have said to yourself, "Of course I'm breathing."

It's common to hold your breath when you're concentrating on an activity, such as exercising, or struggling with a simple task, such as opening a lid on a jar. And often, you don't even realize that you're doing it. When you hold your breath, however, you limit oxygen to your muscles just when they need it the most. Because your muscles can't perform to their capacity without adequate oxygen, you become more easily fatigued.

To keep from holding your breath, exhale when you exert the most energy, such as twisting a jar lid or lifting a heavy box from the floor. Your body will naturally respond by breathing air in.

Pushing

- Bend your knees so your arms are level with the object.
- Maintain normal spine curves and walk, using your legs to push the object ahead of you.

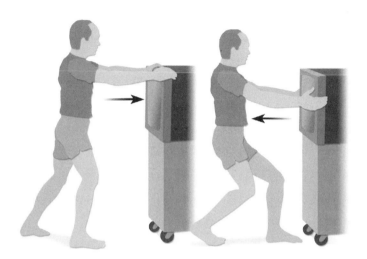

Pulling

- Bend your knees so your arms are level with the object.
- Maintain normal spine curves and walk backward, pulling the object with your whole body weight instead of just your arms or back.
- If possible, push rather than pull.

Using long-handled tools

- Use a rocking motion. With the forward stroke, shift your body weight to your forward foot. When you pull back, shift your weight to your back foot.
- Use arm and leg movements instead of back movements.
- Avoid overreaching and twisting, and use long, smooth strokes.
- Occasionally switch hand positions, exchanging your top hand with your bottom hand.

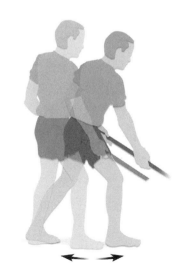

Avoiding temperature extremes

Controlling your environment to avoid extreme heat or cold also can help reduce fatigue. If you need to be outside in hot weather, try to complete your activity early in the morning when the heat and humidity may be less. Wear light-colored clothing to reflect the sun's rays and, if possible, work in an area where there's shade or a breeze.

In cold weather, dress warmly and wear a hat to prevent escape of your body heat. Wear several layers of clothing so you can add or remove layers as needed to maintain a comfortable body temperature.

Chapter 8

Dealing With Your Emotions and Behaviors

When chronic pain intrudes on your life, you may find yourself overwhelmed by intense, often negative, emotions. Panic, grief and anger are just a sampling. Like the pain that spawns them, these emotions can linger and transform you into a different person. A person you don't like. A person no one likes.

Changes in your character, expressed through your words and actions, can damage your sense of self-worth and your relationships. These emotions can also produce changes in your body which sap your energy and intensify your pain.

Now the good news. There are healthful ways for dealing with your inevitable and understandable negative emotions. And if you take advantage of these techniques, you have every reason to expect that you'll develop a stronger character, improve your relationships and become more effective at managing your pain.

Admitting your loss

For many people, the first step in dealing with negative feelings is to admit that the feelings exist. That's very difficult for some people to do, especially in a culture that often praises the optimist and criticizes the complainer.

If you're grappling with chronic pain, one of the earliest and most wrenching emotions you experience is a deep sense of loss. You may miss:
- The healthy person you once were
- Your independence
- Your privacy
- Job satisfaction
- An enjoyable hobby
- Sexual intimacy
- Untroubled family relationships
- Gatherings with friends
- Feelings of energy and confidence
- A sense of happiness

These are difficult losses. You may feel as if you've lost nearly everything precious to you. Your natural response is to grieve.

Feelings associated with grieving

Grieving can trigger various feelings. Even within a single day you may experience several different emotions. Many people respond to chronic pain with the same feelings that often accompany loss of a loved one.

Depression. You become overwhelmed by feelings of sadness, worthlessness and helplessness. You don't feel like doing anything, and you have difficulty concentrating. You withdraw from others.

Anger or frustration. You've tried numerous ways to control your pain and nothing seems to be working. You find yourself more irritable more often. You get upset that others don't seem to understand what you're going through.

Guilt and shame. You sense you're not the person you used to be. You feel you're letting down those who are closest to you.

Denial. You may deny you're in pain. You continually seek "a cure" even though you've been told your pain is incurable.

Acceptance. You stop focusing on things you can't change and begin to look to the future. You accept that your pain is a part of your life.

As you work your way through these emotions, consider these suggestions:
- Recognize your losses as serious. Don't trivialize them.
- Admit your feelings to yourself and others—especially supportive family, friends and your doctor. Acknowledging and talking about your feelings is the first step toward emotional health.
- Give yourself time for emotional healing, and ask your doctor, a counselor or a therapist for advice and help.

Managing your anger

Unrelenting pain, interrupted sleep, unsuccessful treatments, job woes and insurance battles—there are a lot of things that can make you angry when you're in pain.

It's natural to get angry about such experiences. But it's unhealthy to stay angry, bottle up your anger or express it with explosive outbursts.

Mismanaged anger can hurt you in many ways. Whether it's short-term and intense or lingering and subdued, anger causes your body to release chemicals that can lead to headaches, backaches, high blood pressure, irritable bowel syndrome and other health problems. Anger also can influence your pain. It typically produces muscle tension, making it difficult to relax.

Here are some ideas to help you manage your anger:

Identify your anger triggers. If, for example, a visiting friend generally manages to rile you, knowing this ahead of time can help you prepare for the next visit. Think about discussion topics that spark your anger, and practice what to say to defuse the situation. For example, if your friend starts to bring up a past dispute, you might respond by saying, "Oh, we've discussed that before. Certainly we've got more interesting things to talk about."

Identify symptoms of emerging anger. What do you do when you start to get angry? Do you clench your teeth? Do your neck and shoulders begin to tense up? Read these symptoms like a caution light—a warning that you're getting angry.

Respond to your symptoms. When you find yourself becoming angry, take a short time-out. Count to 10, take a few deep breaths, look out a window—anything to buy time so your brain can catch up with your emotions and you can think before you act.

Give yourself time to cool down. Before you confront the person who's made you angry, find a way to release some of your emotional energy. Go for a walk, run or clean the house.

Don't bottle up your anger. If your anger stems from what someone did or said, talk directly to that person. Don't verbally attack the person with accusations and a history of how this person has angered you in the past. Deal only with this episode, and approach it from the perspective of how you feel instead of what the person did. For example, try a statement like this: "I feel hurt by what you said." That way, you're more likely to find a receptive listener than if you launched a blame-offensive statement, such as "You insulted me for the 20th time today!"

Find release valves. Look for creative ways to release the energy produced by your anger. These might include listening to music, painting or writing in your journal.

Seek advice. If anger-provoking situations continue, confide in people who care about you, such as a family member or friend. Ask them to help you brainstorm possible solutions. You might even try role-playing scenes that spark your anger, so you can practice a healthful response.

You can't keep yourself from getting angry, but you can manage your anger so it doesn't become an ongoing problem that aggravates your pain.

Practicing positive thinking

There are many ways to cope with the upsetting changes and emotions chronic pain can produce. One coping technique that many people find effective is positive self-talk. Self-talk is the endless stream of thoughts that run through your head every day. Some people refer to this process as "automatic thinking."

Your automatic thoughts may be positive or negative. Some are based on logic and reason. Others may be misconceptions that you formulate from lack of adequate information. The goal of positive self-talk is to weed out the misconceptions and challenge them with rational and positive thoughts. Studies show that a positive, hopeful attitude can help manage stress, whereas a negative attitude can aggravate it. People who focus on the negative and on their inability to control their chronic pain are more likely to become depressed and physically inactive than those with a positive attitude.

Turning negatives into positives

How can you learn positive self-talk? The process is simple, but it takes time and practice. Throughout the day, stop and evaluate what you're thinking. And find a way to put a positive spin on your negative thoughts. One reasonable rule about self-talk is this: Don't say to yourself any-thing you wouldn't say to someone else. Be gentle and encouraging. If a negative thought enters your mind, evaluate it rationally and respond with affirmations of what is good about yourself.

Eventually, your self-talk will automatically do the same. Your spon-taneous thoughts will become more positive and rational.

Here are some examples:

Negative/irrational beliefs	Positive/rational beliefs
Because of my pain, I'm no longer the person I was. I'm no longer loved and appreciated.	I'm worthy of love, and I'm worthy of being appreciated for all that I am.
People reject me because they can see I'm disabled.	I'm not disabled. I have goals and dreams, and there are many things I can do.
I can't do all that I used to. I'm no longer competent or adequate.	I can do much of what I want to. As long as I don't overdo, I can be actively involved in life.
I have no control over my happiness. Pain controls me.	I can control my happiness. I can be happy and enjoy life regardless of pain.
I used to be able to do so many things. Now I can't do anything.	I can do a lot more than I thought. Almost everything I used to do I can still do to some degree.
If I go out with friends and my pain acts up, I won't be able to manage. I'll embarrass myself and ruin things for everyone.	I can enjoy friends and have a good time. I may take breaks from my usual activities, but it can still be fun.
People at work are upset with me. I have restrictions and they think I'm not doing my share of the work.	I will do the best job I can. My coworkers will have to learn to accept my limitations.
Medical science can do so much. Certainly there must be a cure for my pain.	Medical science can't fix everything. Many medical problems aren't cured but controlled.

Types of distorted thinking

Here are some common forms of negative, irrational thinking. Try to identify and challenge these thoughts:

Filtering. You magnify the negative aspects of a situation and filter out all the positive ones. For example, you had a great day at work. You completed your tasks ahead of time and were complimented for your speedy and thorough work. But you forgot one minor step. That evening you focus only on your oversight and forget about the compliments paid you.

Personalizing. When something bad occurs, you automatically think that you're to blame. For example, you hear that a family picnic has been canceled and you start thinking the change in plans is because no one wanted to be around you.

Generalizing. You see a troubling event as the beginning of an unending cycle. When your pain failed to go away, your thoughts may have proceeded as follows: "I'll never be able to do what I used to." "I'm a burden to everyone around me." "I'm worthless."

Catastrophizing. You automatically anticipate the worst. You refuse to go out with friends for fear your pain will act up and you'll make a fool of yourself. Or, one change in your daily routine leads you to think the day will be a disaster.

Polarizing. You see things only as black and white, good or bad. There's no middle ground. You feel you have to be perfect or you're a failure.

Emotionalizing. With this type of distorted thinking you allow your feelings to control your judgment. If you feel stupid and boring, then you must be stupid and boring.

Challenging your expectations

Some people are perfectionists, constantly striving for excellence. These are the homemakers whose house could pass a military white-glove inspection, the master welders who pride themselves on their precision work and the grandparents who never miss their grandchild's soccer games.

This compulsive perfectionism isn't the lifestyle for someone with chronic pain. Trying to live up to a perfectionist's expectations can become emotionally and physically damaging.

Before pain invaded your life, perhaps you could work 50 to 60 hours a week with no problem, clean your entire house in 2 hours and play a set of tennis every Saturday. Now, even part-time work leaves you exhausted, household chores become intimidating day-long projects and tennis is unimaginable.

As long as you compare yourself with how things used to be, you'll feel miserable about your performance. Your work won't be good enough and your leisure time won't be enjoyable enough.

There is, however, a way to keep an upbeat outlook: Become a perfectionist at adjusting your goals. People who don't adapt to new challenges are more likely to become discouraged and depressed. But those who are flexible enough to adjust their expectations generally have a positive attitude about life and manage to stay active. "I can't work a full-time job and still keep a perfect house," you might say to yourself, "but I can at least clean up the dirty dishes in the kitchen and make sure the floors aren't littered with newspapers and clothes."

Whatever new projects you take on or goals you set for yourself, don't focus on only the outcome. Learn to enjoy the process, not just completion of the task. Look at it as an opportunity to learn and grow.

Learning to assert yourself

Responding to all the challenges of daily life can be difficult. And sometimes, one of the toughest tasks is learning to say no, even when doing so is in your best interest. To keep from disappointing others, you do things you know you shouldn't. You spend all day on your feet shopping with a friend. You agree to stay late at work to finish a last-minute project. This is passive behavior. You put your thoughts, feelings and health aside for the sake of others. Passive behavior can stem from your upbringing and your beliefs about the importance of helping others and treating them with respect. Or, it can result from low self-esteem.

Unfortunately, passive behavior and chronic pain can be a dangerous combination. When you continually give in to the wishes of others—at your expense—your frustration can grow, your self-esteem erode and your pain increase.

Aggressive behavior isn't any better. Contrary to passive behavior, aggressive behavior is being insensitive to others or accomplishing your goals at their expense. Examples include voicing your opinions in such a way that you intimidate others from speaking up, or barging ahead of people who are waiting patiently. This type of behavior can lower your self-respect, alienate relationships and leave you lonely.

So, how do you stand up for yourself without being blunt or hurtful to others? The answer is assertive behavior. Assertive behavior is honestly and openly expressing your feelings while at the same time showing concern for the feelings of others.

Here's an example: "I miss spending time with all of you and I'd like to go with the group golfing. But instead of playing 18 holes, I'm going to bow out after 9 and wait for you to finish. I hope you can understand."

Assertive behavior is based on "I" statements. (The word "I" is used four times in the previous paragraph.) "I" statements allow you to tell people exactly how you feel and what you think, without placing blame or creating feelings of guilt.

Steps to being more assertive

These suggestions can help you be more assertive when communicating with others:

Observe your behavior. Honestly evaluate your behavior when speaking with others. Are there times when you're assertive, such as when communicating with a certain coworker or family member, or are you always passive or aggressive?

Make a mental note of those situations in which you feel you responded well, and those in which you feel you could have done better.

Think before you respond. When you want to make a statement or you're asked a question, think briefly about the best way to get your point across assertively, instead of simply blurting out an automatic response.

Plan for a difficult situation. Think about a situation you're likely to encounter in which you'll need to be assertive. Close your eyes and imagine how you'll respond. What might the person say? What will you say in return?

Here's an example. Your company is making plans to launch a new product and you know your boss is going to ask you to head up the launch committee because you can never say no. But you're having trouble keeping up with your duties as it is, and you know the stress and long days involved to get the product ready would be difficult.

Picture your boss walking into your office and sitting in the chair by your desk. When your boss says, "I'd really like you to take on this assignment," practice your response: "I understand the importance of this project. However, my schedule is already very full and I need to keep from overextending myself. If there is another way I can help that doesn't require as much time, I'm happy to do it."

Pay attention to your body language. As you practice being more assertive, observe how you stand or sit, along with your gestures, facial expressions and eye contact. For example, when talking to someone, do you look at the person? Or do you stare at the ceiling or floor or out a window?

Boosting your self-esteem

Your struggle with chronic pain can result in some damaging blows to your self-image. Some of these are self-imposed, such as your inability to measure up to your own expectations. Others may come from family, friends, colleagues or even strangers. Perhaps they criticize or ignore you because you don't meet their standards or because you look haggard from your struggle with pain.

It's important to maintain a strong sense of self-worth. The better you feel about yourself, the better you'll take care of yourself. In addition, a positive self-image has been linked to a stronger immune system. So, feeling good about yourself may actually improve your health.

Many of the steps discussed in this chapter—managing your anger, practicing positive thinking, challenging your expectations and learning to assert yourself—will have a positive effect on your self-esteem. As you learn how to control and express your emotions, you'll feel better about yourself and more confident in your abilities, and your self-image will improve.

There may be days, however, when your self-esteem could use a little energizing. When that happens, consider these suggestions:

Structure your day with goals you can meet. When the day is done, you'll feel a sense of accomplishment.

Talk with a friend. Having someone who's willing to take time to listen to you lets you know that you're valued.

Spend time with others. It will make you feel more connected and less alone.

Help someone. It reminds you that your life makes a difference.

Treat yourself to something you enjoy. This might be some new music, a great book or a scoop of gourmet ice cream. Just as you buy gifts for others who are feeling blue, you need to do the same for yourself.

Spruce up your appearance. Try a different hairstyle. Buy some new clothes. The better you look, the better you feel about yourself.

List reasons people like you. It reminds you that you have special qualities people enjoy.

List things you do well. Then do one of them.

Chapter 9

Managing Life's Stresses

Just as with your emotions and behaviors, pain and stress go hand in hand. When you're in pain, you're less able to handle everyday "stressors." Common hassles turn into major obstacles. Stress also causes you to do things that intensify your pain, such as tense your muscles, grit your teeth and stiffen your shoulders. In short, pain causes stress, and stress intensifies pain.

The first step in breaking this pain-stress cycle is to realize that stress is your response to an event, not the event itself. It's something you can control. That's why events that are stressful for some people aren't for others. For example, your morning commute may leave you anxious and tense because you use it as worry time. Your coworker, however, finds his commute relaxing. He enjoys his time alone without distractions. Understanding that you have control over your stress can help you develop positive strategies for dealing with stress.

How you respond to stress

When you encounter stress, your body responds in a manner similar to a physical threat. It automatically gears up to face the challenge ("fight") or musters enough strength to move out of trouble's way ("flight"). This "fight-or-flight" response results from the release of hormones that cause your body to shift into overdrive. Your heart beats faster, your blood pressure increases and your breathing quickens and becomes more shallow. Your nervous system also springs into action, causing your facial muscles to tighten and your body to perspire more.

Stress can be negative or positive:

- Positive stress provides a feeling of excitement and opportunity. Among athletes, positive stress often helps them perform better in competition than in practice. Other examples of positive stress include a new job or birth of a child.
- Negative stress occurs when you feel out of control or under constant or intense pressure. You may have trouble concentrating, or you may feel alone. Family, finances, work, isolation and health problems, including pain, are common causes of negative stress.

The danger of ongoing negative stress is its effect on your body. Tightening of your muscles, anxiety and nervousness contribute to your pain.

In addition, stress is thought to play a role in several illnesses. When your heart rate increases, you become at greater risk for development of chest pain (angina) and irregularities in your heart rhythm (arrhythmia). Surges in your heart rate and blood pressure also can trigger a heart attack or damage your heart muscle or coronary arteries. The hormone cortisol released during stress may suppress your immune system, making you more susceptible to infections and disease. Stress also can cause headaches and worsen intestinal problems and asthma.

What are your triggers?

Stress often is associated with situations or events that you find difficult to handle. How you view things also affects your level of stress. If you have unrealistic or high expectations, chances are you'll experience more than your fair share of stress.

Take some time to think about what causes you stress. Your stress may be linked to external factors, such as:

- Work
- Family
- Community
- Environment
- Unpredictable events

Stress also can come from internal factors, such as:

- Unrealistic or high expectations

- Perfectionism
- Negative attitudes and feelings
- Irresponsible behavior
- Poor health habits

Jot down what seem to be sources of stress for you. And then ask yourself if there's anything you can do to lessen or avoid them. Some stressors you can control, whereas other events in life you can't.

Concentrate on events you can change. For situations that are beyond your control, look for ways to adapt—to remain calm under trying circumstances.

Strategies for reducing stress

It's one thing to be aware of stress in your daily life, but it's another to know how to change it. As you look through your list of stressors, think carefully about why they're so bothersome. For example, if your busy day is a source of stress, ask yourself if it's because you tend to squeeze too many things into your day or because you aren't organized.

The following techniques can help you reduce those sources of stress you can control and better cope with those you can't.

Change your lifestyle

Consider these changes to your normal routine:

Plan your day. This can help you feel more in control of your life. You might start by getting up 15 minutes earlier to ease the morning rush. Do unpleasant tasks early in the day and be done with them. Keep a written schedule of your daily activities so you're not faced with conflicts or last-minute rushes to get to an appointment or activity on time. Because a pain flare-up can happen at any time, have a backup plan—decide what you can manage now and what can wait until later.

Simplify your schedule. Prioritize, plan and pace yourself. Learn to delegate responsibility to others at home and at work. Say "no" to added responsibilities or commitments if you're not up to doing them. And don't feel guilty if you aren't productive every waking moment.

Get organized. Organize your home and work space so that you know where things are and can easily reach them. Keep your house, car and personal belongings in working order to prevent untimely, expensive and stressful repairs.

Take occasional breaks. Take time to relax, stretch or walk periodically during the day.

Exercise regularly. Regular physical activity helps loosen your muscles and relieves your emotional intensity. Try to exercise for a total of at least 30 minutes most days of the week.

Get enough sleep. This can give you the energy you need to face each day. Going to sleep and awakening at a consistent time also may help you sleep more soundly.

Eat well. A diet that includes a variety of foods provides the right mix of nutrients to keep your body systems working well. When you're healthy, you're better able to control stress and pain.

Change the pace. Occasionally break away from your routine and explore new territory without a schedule. Take a vacation, even if it's just a weekend get-away.

Be positive. There's no room for "Yes, but...." Avoiding negative self-talk can be difficult. It helps to spend time with people who have a positive outlook, take themselves lightly or have a sense of humor. Laughter actually helps ease pain. It releases endorphins, chemicals in your brain that give you a sense of well-being.

Stay connected. Recognize when you need the support of family and friends. Talking about your problems with others can often relieve pent-up emotions and lead to solutions you hadn't thought of on your own.

Be patient. Realizing that improvements in your health may take time can help reduce anxiety and stress.

SOLVE your problems

Problem solving is a coping skill that can help you manage everyday difficulties that may seem overwhelming. Problem-solving skills can help you assess a situation and respond effectively and productively. Developing these skills will help you view problems as challenges that you can overcome, rather than threats you should avoid.

The letters in the word "SOLVE" will help you remember a useful five-step problem-solving strategy*:

State the problem. The first step is to identify what the problem is. What's bothering you? What are you concerned about? Ask yourself if your evaluation of your problem is objective and on target.

---

*The SOLVE strategy is modified from Self-Management Training Program for Chronic Headache: Patient Manual, Volume II, by Donald Penzien, Ph.D., and Jeanette Rains, Ph.D. (This information was obtained from Jamison RN: Learning to Master Your Chronic Pain. Sarasota, FL: Professional Resource Press, 1996. By permission of Professional Resource Exchange.)

Outline the problem. Break the problem down and define the specifics. Ask yourself these questions: Who is involved? Where and when does it happen? What precedes it? What happens next? How do I react? What role do I play? The idea is not to punish yourself, but to determine what part of the problem you can actually solve.

List possible solutions. Decide what you want out of the situation. Consider what you don't want to happen, and what needs to happen for things to get back on track. Brainstorm ways to solve your problem. Be creative and consider all your options, even the most unlikely or unusual ones. See if you can group any of your ideas—sometimes a combination of alternatives is the best solution.

View the consequences. Once you've made your list, look at the pros and cons for each option. What will happen if you choose a particular solution? How will it make you feel? What impact will it have on others? Will it help you reach your goal? What are the short-term and long-term consequences? What prevents you from carrying this out? How much time, money and energy will it take? Do the benefits outweigh the costs? Now rank the alternatives and choose the option that promises the best outcome.

Execute your solution. Once you've devised your plan, rehearse your strategies. Try out your solution and then evaluate it. Revise and rework your plan until you feel comfortable with it.

Relief through relaxation

You can't avert all sources of stress, such as an unexpected visit from family or friends or a problem at work. However, you can modify how you react to these situations by practicing relaxation techniques. Relaxation helps relieve stress that can aggravate chronic pain. It also helps prevent muscle spasms and reduces muscle tension.

Relaxation won't cure your pain, but it can:
- Reduce anxiety and conserve energy
- Increase your self-control when dealing with a stressful situation
- Help you recognize the difference between tense muscles and relaxed ones
- Help you physically and emotionally handle your daily demands
- Help you remain alert, energetic and productive

Keep in mind, though, that the benefits of relaxation are only as good as your efforts. Learning to relax takes time.

Techniques to try

There are many ways to relax, so pick one that works best for you.

Deep breathing. Unlike children, most adults breathe from their chest. Each time you breathe in your chest expands, and each time you

Taking a breather

Here's an exercise to help you practice deep, relaxed breathing. Rehearse it throughout the day until it becomes natural so that you can automatically apply it when you feel stressed.

- Sit comfortably with your feet flat on the floor.
- Loosen tight clothing around your abdomen and waist.
- Place your hands in your lap or at your side.
- Breathe in slowly (through your nose if possible) while counting to 4. Allow your abdomen to expand as you breathe in.
- Pause for a second and then exhale at a normal rate through your mouth

If you can't feel your abdomen expand as you breathe in:

- Gently push your abdomen with your hand as you breathe out.
- Allow your abdomen to expand against your hand as you breathe in.

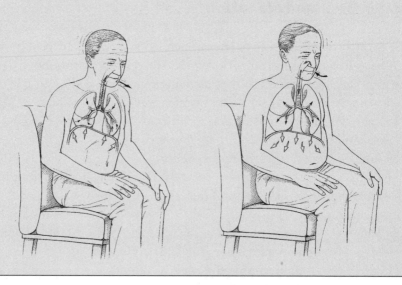

breathe out it contracts. Children, however, generally breathe from their diaphragm, the muscle that separates the chest from the abdomen. Deep breathing from your diaphragm—which adults can relearn—is relaxing. It also exchanges more carbon dioxide for oxygen, to give you more energy.

You can use deep breathing as your only means of relaxation or as a warm-up and cool-down method for other techniques (see "Taking a breather").

Progressive muscle relaxation. This technique involves relaxing a series of muscles one at a time. First, raise the tension level in a group of muscles, such as a leg or arm, by tightening the muscles and then relaxing them. Concentrate on letting the tension go in each muscle. Then move on to the next muscle group. Be careful, however, not to over-tense muscles near your pain sites.

Word repetition. Choose a word or phrase that is a cue for you to relax, and then constantly repeat it. While repeating the word or phrase, try to breathe deeply and slowly and think of something that gives you pleasant sensations of warmth and heaviness.

Guided imagery. Also known as visualization, this method of relaxation involves lying quietly and picturing yourself in a pleasant and peaceful setting. You experience the setting with all of your senses as if you were actually there. For instance, imagine lying on the beach. Picture the beautiful blue sky, smell the saltwater, hear the waves and feel the warm breeze on your skin. The messages your brain receives as you experience these senses help you to relax.

Tips to help you succeed

No matter what relaxation method you choose, these simple steps can help you be successful:

Practice. If relaxation is new to you, you may not notice immediate benefits. In fact, you may feel uncomfortable at first.

Work on your relaxation skills at least once or twice a day until they come naturally. When you're just beginning, a quiet place and a relaxation tape

More ways to relax

In this chapter we talk about some basic relaxation techniques. Other methods for reducing or relieving stress include meditation, yoga, hypnosis and biofeedback. We discuss these relaxation techniques in Chapter 13 (page 133).

often help. But work toward relaxing without a tape so you can do it anywhere, anytime.

Get comfortable. Loosen tight clothing, and remove your shoes and belt, if need be.

Vary your schedule. Practice relaxation at different times throughout the day. The idea is to learn how to relax whenever you need to.

Be patient. A wandering mind is normal when you start out. Just keep bringing your attention back to relaxation. And don't worry about how well you're doing. It takes practice for this skill to become automatic.

Some cues you're relaxed are feelings of being tingly, warm, comfortable, heavy, light, or feeling as if you're floating.

Chapter 10

Interacting With Family and Friends

As trying as chronic pain is to you, it can be every bit as troubling to your family and friends. They want to help you, but they may not know how. So, they say or do things they think are helpful, but may only add to your frustration.

Because chronic pain is such a personal experience, it's difficult for family and friends to understand exactly what you're feeling and going through. No one knows your pain like you. In addition, when pain takes over, communication often suffers. You may not feel like discussing your pain or problems related to it. And family and friends may hesitate to approach certain subjects for fear they will anger or frustrate you.

You need family and friends to help you manage your pain and move on with your life. But they can help you only if you help them.

Benefits of social interaction

People with a solid support system have many health advantages over people without support. For example, people with caring family and friends generally:
- Cope better with chronic pain
- Are less likely to experience depression
- Are more independent
- Recover faster from illness
- Have a stronger immune system

- Have lower blood pressure
- Have lower cholesterol
- Live longer

Through your own experiences, you may know what researchers are talking about. You've felt how quickly a cup of coffee with a neighbor has lifted your spirits. You've experienced how a helping hand from a relative has helped you get through a "bad" day. And you know how even a short trip out with a friend can invigorate you. Being around others can temporarily help you forget about your frustrations.

Developing a strong support system

Good friends and a supportive family can provide encouraging words, offer gentle but helpful criticisms and lend a hand when you need assistance. Family and friends also help replace sadness with smiles and laughter. In this way, they contribute to your health and well-being.

Making friendships and maintaining family ties seem to come more naturally for some people than for others. But even if you're not an outgoing person, you need social support. If your support system is in need of a little strengthening, try these suggestions:

- Answer phone calls and letters.
- Accept invitations to events, even if it feels awkward and difficult at first.
- Don't wait to be invited somewhere. Take the initiative and call someone.
- Set aside past differences and approach your relationships with a clean slate.
- Take part in community organizations, neighborhood events or family get-togethers.
- Strike up a conversation with the person next to you at a local gathering. You could be introducing yourself to a new friend.
- Talk about things that other people are interested in. And be an alert listener.
- Don't give up on existing relationships.

Good relationships require patience, compromise and acceptance. Without these things, the relationship can become a source of stress instead of support. Family and friends need to learn to accept you along with your needs, and you need to accept them along with theirs.

How does your social network stack up?
A strong support system is associated with better health and a longer life. Check each statement that is true about your relationships. Each statement marks an important link in your social network.

_____ I have friends or family members nearby to help me.
_____ I'm involved in a community or religious organization.
_____ I have at least one friend or relative that I can talk to about almost anything.
_____ I keep in daily contact with other people.

Statements you didn't mark are areas you might work on to improve your support system.

It's true that relationships can sometimes be difficult. Your friends and family may want more of your time and energy than you can spare. But instead of drawing away from those you're close to, educate them about your pain. And allow friends and family members to tell you how your pain has affected them.

This will help those closest to you understand why you may not always be able to keep up with them or do all of the things they ask. It will also help you understand how your pain affects others.

Improving your communication skills

Discussing your thoughts and feelings can be difficult even in the best of times. With chronic pain, the task doesn't get any easier. Instead of continually telling people what you're going through and how you're feeling, it's often easier to withdraw or say as little as possible.

The problem with this tactic, however, is that it frustrates and alienates your family and friends. Communication is the glue that holds your relationships together. Without honest communication flowing freely in both directions, misunderstanding and resentment swell.

So how do you improve communication?

Express what you're feeling. The only way people can begin to understand what you're thinking or feeling is if you tell them. But do it in a positive manner, not one in which you appear to be whining or accusatory. Negative emotions only increase your chances for a negative response.

For example, if you're frustrated because your friends don't include you in their activities anymore you might say, "I miss spending time with you on Saturdays and I sure would like to join you in softball or bicycling." Your friends may incorrectly assume that you can't take part in recreational events. That's why they don't invite you to join them, not because they don't want to be around you.

Don't lie about your pain. Close family and friends may know not to ask how you're doing every time they see you. But some people won't understand that you may always have some degree of pain. When they inquire how you're doing, don't pretend it doesn't hurt. But don't exaggerate your pain, either. You might respond, "I still have pain, but I'm learning to manage it."

Ask for help when you need it. You were probably taught to cherish your independence, so it may be difficult for you to ask for help. But sometimes you need help. Try asking in a way that explains what's going on. For example: "I've invited friends over for dinner and it's taking me longer to get the meal prepared than I anticipated. I look forward to having friends come, but I need some help. Could you please come over and lend me a hand for a while?"

Be a cheerful receiver. When someone helps you or gives you a heartfelt compliment about your progress, say "Thanks." Don't feel depressed that you needed the help or the emotional boost.

Discuss communication roadblocks. If the flow of communication between you and a family member or friend becomes one-sided, talk about it. Set aside your pride for a while, and take the risk of saying exactly how you feel. If that fails to open the channel, don't give up too soon. Consider asking advice from a counselor.

Put your toughest communication problems in writing. Use your journal to express those feelings you have trouble communicating. This not only will buy you some time to let these feelings settle but also will give you practice in expressing them when you're ready to discuss them.

Ways family and friends can help

Chances are your family and friends have asked you what they can do to help you. And, perhaps, you didn't know what to say, or you felt guilty admitting you needed any type of special treatment. Or, maybe, they've decided to "help" in ways that irritate you more than anything else. They think they're doing things to make you feel better, but they're not.

When people ask you how they can help, tell them. Here are some suggestions you might pass along:

Learn more about my pain. Chronic pain is difficult to understand. Reading about it will help family and friends better understand what you're going through, how they can help and when they shouldn't help. For instance, continually doing tasks for you that you can do for yourself unintentionally contributes to your loss of independence and self-confidence.

Don't let conversations always gravitate to my pain. It's easy for friends and family to get caught up in discussing your pain. But that only reminds you of your condition and draws attention to your pain—something you're trying to avoid.

Try not to hover over me. Being overly attentive to someone with persistent pain can actually interfere with rehabilitation. One study found that people with chronic pain who were observed by an overly attentive spouse reported more pain than when they were observed by someone else.

Tell your spouse or partner that you appreciate the concern, but that he or she doesn't need to be your butler. To manage your pain, you need to learn to do things for yourself again. Many studies confirm that when family members, in particular, are supportive in upbeat and healthful ways that don't reinforce pain behaviors, such as limping, groaning or grimacing, the person with chronic pain has a much better prognosis.

Join me in activities. Having friends and family members accompany you for a walk or go with you to support group meetings or doctor visits offers many benefits. It gives you a chance to talk and share time together. It also gives them an opportunity to learn more about your need to exercise and stay active.

Don't give up things you enjoy for my sake. Those closest to you may consciously or unconsciously change their lifestyle because of your pain. But that doesn't encourage you and it may make you feel guilty. For example, if you and a friend enjoyed fishing together, don't let your friend sell his poles just because he thinks you can't fish anymore. You may not be able to fish from dawn to dusk as you used to, but you can fish for a few hours.

Be available to listen to me. Sometimes you simply need someone to listen. A family member or friend who can lend emotional support like this provides a release valve for your daily stresses. People with chronic pain who feel they have the support of loved ones seem to cope better with their pain, return to work sooner and live more active lives.

As they listen, your family members and friends can help you by reminding you of the progress you're making and keeping you focused on positive solutions to your problems.

Take care of yourself. Your pain, and worrying about you, can take a toll on friends and family members. They, too, can experience worry, depression and exhaustion. It's important that those you care about take care of their health as well. Just as you need their support, they need yours.

Chapter 11

Caring for Yourself and Your Health

L iving well with chronic pain isn't just about steps to control your pain. It's about caring for your overall health, so you can enjoy life to its fullest.

We've already discussed many issues that are important to good health, such as improving your physical fitness, reducing stress and learning to relax. In this chapter, we focus on other factors that also can help you stay active and productive and feel good about yourself.

Getting a good night's sleep

Sleep refreshes you. It improves your attitude and gives you energy for physical activity and to fight off fatigue and stress. It also boosts your immune system, reducing your risk for illness.

If you aren't sleeping well, it may be because your pain is keeping you from falling asleep or is waking you up at night. Other conditions that also can interfere with sleep are:

- Stress
- Anxiety
- Depression
- Alcohol
- Stimulant medications
- Regular use of over-the-counter sleeping pills

- Lack of physical activity
- Change in your environment
- Poor sleep habits

To improve your sleep, it's important to recognize factors that may be contributing to your restless nights.

Stages of sleep

There are two types of sleep—rapid eye movement (REM) and nonrapid eye movement (NREM). NREM is divided into three phases: light sleep, intermediate sleep and deep sleep (see "Your Natural Sleep Cycle").

Throughout the night you continually move from one phase of sleep to another. REM sleep is a period of increased activity. This is the phase of sleep during which you dream and your body functions, such as your heart rate, blood pressure and breathing, increase. During NREM sleep your brain activity decreases and these functions slow.

Deep sleep is the most restful kind of sleep. It's also the phase of sleep many people with chronic pain miss. If you have trouble falling asleep, frequently awaken at night or wake up feeling as though you haven't slept at all, you may not be reaching periods of deep sleep. Instead, you spend your night in light or intermediate sleep. Intermediate sleep helps refresh your body, but it doesn't provide the relaxation and energy boost you receive from deep sleep.

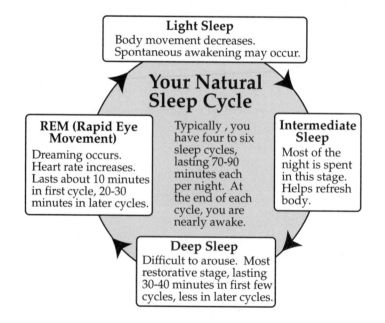

Light Sleep
Body movement decreases.
Spontaneous awakening may occur.

Your Natural Sleep Cycle

REM (Rapid Eye Movement)
Dreaming occurs. Heart rate increases. Lasts about 10 minutes in first cycle, 20-30 minutes in later cycles.

Typically, you have four to six sleep cycles, lasting 70-90 minutes each per night. At the end of each cycle, you are nearly awake.

Intermediate Sleep
Most of the night is spent in this stage. Helps refresh body.

Deep Sleep
Difficult to arouse. Most restorative stage, lasting 30-40 minutes in first few cycles, less in later cycles.

Strategies to help you sleep better
Before bed, take time to relax. That might include:
- Practicing relaxation techniques
- Taking a warm bath
- Having a light snack
- Reading
- Listening to soothing music
- Writing in your journal

Relaxation helps reduce your pain so you can fall asleep more easily. It also helps you achieve more restful sleep.

Here are other suggestions that may help you sleep better:

Establish regular sleep hours. Go to bed and wake up at the same time each day. Following a regular pattern often improves sleep.

Limit your time in bed. Too much sleep can promote shallow, unrestful sleep. Aim for 8 hours of sleep a night. Some people can get by on just 4 or 5 hours. Others need up to 10 hours a night. Don't stay in bed longer than 10 hours.

Don't "try" to sleep. The harder you try, the more awake you'll become. Read or watch television until you become drowsy and fall asleep naturally.

Limit bedroom activities. Save your bedroom for sleep and sex. Don't watch TV or take your work materials to bed.

Avoid or limit caffeine, alcohol and nicotine. Caffeine and nicotine can keep you from falling asleep. Alcohol causes unrestful sleep and frequent awakenings.

Minimize interruptions. Close your bedroom door or create a subtle background noise, such as a fan, to drown out other noises. Keep your bedroom temperature comfortable, and drink less before bed so you won't have to get up at night to go to the bathroom.

Keep active. Regular physical activity helps you sleep more soundly. Try to get at least 30 minutes of physical activity daily, preferably 5 to 6 hours before bedtime. Also keep occupied throughout the day. Boredom promotes restless sleep.

Schedule "worry time." Don't take your worries to bed with you. During the evening, address your worries and ways to solve them.

Check your medications. Ask your doctor if they might be contributing to your difficulty sleeping. Also check over-the-counter products to see if they contain caffeine or other stimulants (such as pseudoephedrine).

To nap, or not?

The urge for a mid-day snooze is built into your body's biologic clock. It generally occurs between 1 p.m. and 4 p.m., when your body temperature naturally dips slightly.

Napping isn't a substitute for a full night's sleep. Don't nap if you have trouble sleeping at night. If you find a nap refreshes you and doesn't interfere with nighttime sleep, try these ideas:

Keep it short. Thirty minutes is ideal. Naps longer than 1 to 2 hours are more likely to interfere with your nighttime sleep.

Take a mid-afternoon nap. Naps at this time produce a physically invigorating slumber.

If you can't nap, just rest. Lie down and keep your mind on something relaxing.

What about sleep medications?

If you're having trouble sleeping, your doctor may prescribe a medication until other steps to improve your sleep and control your pain have time to take effect. The downfall of many prescription and over-the-counter sleep medications is they often don't allow you to experience all phases of sleep. The drugs also can lose their effectiveness and cause side effects, including dry mouth, next-day drowsiness and physical dependence. That's why it's best to try to improve your sleep with changes in your lifestyle.

For sleep difficulties associated with chronic pain, antidepressants are often prescribed. A side effect of some antidepressants is drowsiness. When taken before bed, they can help you sleep. Plus, antidepressants aren't addictive.

Controlling your weight

Maintaining a healthy weight reduces your risk for illnesses such as coronary artery disease, high cholesterol, high blood pressure and diabetes. It's also easier to control your pain when you're not overweight. That's because excessive weight saps your energy level, increases stress on your muscles and joints and decreases your flexibility. It's not necessary that you become "thin." But losing even a few pounds may make an improvement in your pain level.

Is your weight healthy?

Three do-it-yourself evaluations can tell you if your weight is healthy or whether you could benefit from weight loss.

Body mass index. Body mass index (BMI) is a formula that considers your weight and your height in determining whether you have a healthful or unhealthful percentage of total body fat. It's a better measurement of health risks related to your weight than using your bathroom scale or standard weight-and-height tables.

To determine your BMI, locate your height on the chart on the next page and follow it across until you reach the weight nearest yours. Look at the top of the column for the BMI rating. (If your weight is less than the weight nearest yours, your BMI may be slightly less. If your weight is greater than the weight nearest yours, your BMI may be slightly greater.) A BMI of 19 to 24 is considered healthy. A BMI of 25 to 29 signifies overweight, and a BMI of 30 or more indicates obesity.

Waist circumference. This measurement indicates where most of your body fat is located. People who carry most of their weight around their waists are often referred to as "apples." Those who carry most of their weight below the waist, around their hips and thighs, are known as "pears."

Generally, it's better to have a pear shape than an apple shape. That's because fat around your abdomen is associated with a greater risk for a heart attack and other weight-related diseases.

To determine whether you're carrying too much weight around your abdomen, measure your waist circumference. Find the highest point on each of your hip bones and measure across your abdomen just above those points. A measurement of more than 40 inches (102 centimeters) in men and 35 inches (88 centimeters) in women signifies increased health risks, especially if you have a BMI of 25 or more.

Personal and family history. An evaluation of your medical history, along with that of your family, is equally important in determining whether your weight is healthy.

Answer these questions:

- Do you have a health condition, such as arthritis or back pain, that would benefit from weight loss?

What's your BMI?

Body mass index (BMI)

BMI	Healthy		Overweight					Obesity				
	19	24	25	26	27	28	29	30	35	40	45	50
Height						Weight in pounds						
4'10"	91	115	119	124	129	134	138	143	167	191	215	239
4'11"	94	119	124	128	133	138	143	148	173	198	222	247
5'0"	97	123	128	133	138	143	148	153	179	204	230	255
5'1"	100	127	132	137	143	148	153	158	185	211	238	264
5'2"	104	131	136	142	147	153	158	164	191	218	246	273
5'3"	107	135	141	146	152	158	163	169	197	225	254	282
5'4"	110	140	145	151	157	163	169	174	204	232	262	291
5'5"	114	144	150	156	162	168	174	180	210	240	270	300
5'6"	118	148	155	161	167	173	179	186	216	247	278	309
5'7"	121	153	159	166	172	178	185	191	223	255	287	319
5'8"	125	158	164	171	177	184	190	197	230	262	295	328
5'9"	128	162	169	176	182	189	196	203	236	270	304	338
5'10"	132	167	174	181	188	195	202	209	243	278	313	348
5'11"	136	172	179	186	193	200	208	215	250	286	322	358
6'0"	140	177	184	191	199	206	213	221	258	294	331	368
6'1"	144	182	189	197	204	212	219	227	265	302	340	378
6'2"	148	186	194	202	210	218	225	233	272	311	350	389
6'3"	152	192	200	208	216	224	232	240	279	319	359	399
6'4"	156	197	205	213	221	230	238	246	287	328	369	410

Modified from National Institutes of Health Clinical Guidelines on the Identification, Evaluation, and Treatment of Overweight and Obesity in Adults, 1998.

- Do you have a family history of a weight-related illness, such as diabetes or high blood pressure?
- Have you gained considerable weight since high school? Weight gain in adulthood is associated with increased health risks.
- Do you smoke cigarettes, have more than two alcoholic drinks per day or live with considerable stress? In combination with these behaviors, excess weight can have greater health implications.

Adding up the results. If your BMI shows you aren't overweight, you're not carrying too much weight around your abdomen and you answered "no" to all of the personal or family history questions, there's probably no health advantage to changing your weight. Your weight is healthy.

If your BMI is between 25 and 29, your waist circumference exceeds healthy guidelines or you answered "yes" to at least one personal and family health question, you might benefit from losing a few pounds. Discuss your weight with your doctor during your next checkup.

If your BMI is 30 or more, losing weight will improve your overall health and energy level and reduce your risk for future illness.

Losing weight successfully

The best way to lose weight safely and keep it off permanently is through lifestyle changes. There are many products and programs that promise to help you shed pounds, but they aren't always safe or effective. Once you go off the diet, you gain the weight back again.

Here are some steps that can help you be successful:

Make a commitment. You must be motivated to lose weight because it's what you want, not what someone else wants you to do. Only you can help yourself lose weight. However, that doesn't mean that you have to do everything alone. Your doctor, a registered dietitian or other health care professional can help you develop a plan to lose weight.

Think positively. Don't dwell on what you're giving up to lose weight. Instead, concentrate on what you're gaining. Instead of thinking, "I really miss eating a doughnut for breakfast," tell yourself, "I feel a lot better when I eat whole wheat toast and cereal in the morning."

Get your priorities straight. Timing is critical. Don't try to lose weight if you're distracted by other problems. It takes a lot of mental and physical energy to change habits. If you're having family or financial problems or you're trying to wean yourself from medications, it may not be the best time to try losing weight.

Set a realistic goal. Don't aim for a weight that's unrealistic. Instead, try for a comfortable weight you maintained easily as a young adult. If you've always been overweight, aim for a weight that will help reduce pressure on your joints and muscles and improve your energy level.

Accept that healthful weight loss is slow and steady. A good weight loss plan generally involves losing no more than 1 to 2 pounds (0.5 to 1 kilogram) a week. Set weekly or monthly goals that allow you to check off your successes.

Know your habits. Ask yourself if you tend to eat when you're bored, angry, tired, anxious, depressed or socially pressured. If you do, try these possible solutions:

- Before eating anything, ask yourself if you really want it.
- Do something to distract yourself from your desire to eat, such as telephone a friend or run an errand.
- If you're feeling stressed or angry, direct that energy constructively. Instead of eating, practice a relaxation technique or take a brisk walk.

Don't starve yourself. Liquid meals, diet pills and special food combinations aren't your answer to long-term weight control and better health.

Most people try to lose weight by eating 1,000 to 1,500 calories a day. Cutting calories to fewer than 1,200 if you're a woman or 1,400 if you're a man doesn't provide enough food to keep you satisfied. Plus it promotes temporary loss of fluids and loss of healthy muscle, instead of permanent loss of fat.

The best way to lose weight is to eat more healthful foods.

Get and stay active. Dieting alone will help you lose weight. But by adding 30 minutes of moderate activity most days of the week, you can double your rate of weight loss. Physical activity is the most important factor related to long-term weight loss. It promotes loss of body fat and development of muscle. These changes in body composition help raise the rate at which you burn calories, making it easier to maintain your weight loss.

Think lifelong. It's not enough to eat healthful foods and exercise for a few weeks or even several months. As with other strategies for managing your pain, you have to incorporate these new behaviors into your life.

Eating for better health

Food can't control your pain. But a nutritionally balanced diet can improve the way you feel. In addition to helping you lose weight, eating a variety of foods gives you energy and a sense of well-being. Nutritious foods, combined with a healthy weight, are also your best bet for staying healthy.

Eating well = variety

If you think of eating well as counting calories or tallying fat grams, it's time to think about food in a new way. Eating well means enjoying great taste as well as great nutrition.

No one food provides all the nutrients your body needs. A variety of foods helps ensure the right mix of nutrients for good health.

Here are the types and amounts of foods to try to eat every day. By emphasizing these foods, you limit consumption of fat, saturated fat and cholesterol in your diet.

Grains: 6 to 11 servings. Grains—cereals, breads, rice and pasta— provide a variety of nutrients and are rich in energy-filled complex carbohydrates. Despite a common misconception that breads and pasta are fattening, these foods are low in fat and calories. It's what you put on breads and pastas—spreads and sauces made from fats, oils or cheese— that add calories.

Select whole grains when possible because they contain more dietary fiber than refined grains. Fiber improves blood cholesterol levels and blood sugar control. It also speeds digestion, helping to prevent constipation.

Vegetables: At least 3 servings. Vegetables provide a variety of vitamins, minerals and, in most cases, fiber. In addition, they contain phytochemicals, substances that can reduce your risk of cardiovascular disease and some cancers. Vegetables are also naturally low in calories and virtually fat-free.

Fruits: At least 2 servings. All fruit in any form—fresh, dried, frozen and canned—plays an important role in eating well. Along with few calories and little or no fat, fruit contains vitamins, minerals, phytochemicals and dietary fiber. Plus, fruit serves as natural sweeteners to other foods.

Dairy products: 2 to 3 servings. Milk, yogurt and cheese are outstanding sources of calcium and vitamin D, which helps your body absorb calcium. They also provide protein needed to make and maintain body tissues. However, dairy products can be high in fat and cholesterol, so low-fat or fat-free products are your best choices.

Poultry, seafood and meat: No more than 3 servings. These foods are rich sources of protein, with B vitamins, iron and zinc. However, because even lean varieties contain fat and cholesterol, limit all animal foods.

Determining a serving

The number of servings recommended for each food group may sound like a lot of food. But serving sizes are smaller than you may think. Here are some examples of what counts as 1 serving for these food groups:

Food	Serving examples
Grains	1 slice whole-wheat bread
	½ bagel or English muffin
	½ cup (3 oz./90 g) cooked cereal, rice or pasta
	½ cup (3 oz./30 g) ready-to-eat cereal
Fruits & vegetables	¼ cup (1 ½ oz./46 g) raisins
	¾ cup (6 fl. oz./180 mL) 100% fruit juice
	1 medium apple or banana
	12 grapes
	1 cup (2 oz./60 g) raw leafy green vegetables
	½ cup (3 oz./90 g) cooked vegetables
	1 medium potato
Dairy products	1 cup (8 fl. oz./250 mL) low-fat or fat-free milk
	1 cup (8 oz./250 g) low-fat or fat-free yogurt
	1 ½ oz. (45 g) reduced-fat or fat-free cheese
	2 cups (16 oz./500 g) low-fat or fat-free cottage cheese
Poultry, seafood & meat	2-3 oz. (60-90 g) cooked skinless poultry, seafood or lean meat
Legumes	½ cup (3 ½ oz./105 g) cooked beans, dried peas or lentils

Legumes: Frequently, as alternatives to animal foods. Low in fat and with no cholesterol, legumes—beans, dried peas and lentils—are your best source of plant protein. They also provide nutrients, phytochemicals and dietary fiber.

Fats, sweets and alcohol: Sparingly. Alcohol and the fats and sugars that occur naturally in certain foods provide calories with no nutrients. The most obvious way to cut fat in your diet is to reduce the amount of pure fat—butter, margarine and vegetable oils—you add to food during cooking. Also limit sweets, such as candy, sugar-sweetened soft drinks and desserts.

Limiting alcohol

The best advice about alcohol is: If you drink, do it in moderation (see "What's moderate drinking?"). And if you're taking medication, it might be best not to drink any alcohol.

Alcohol can increase the potency and side effects of many prescription drugs, including pain relievers and antidepressants. In addition, regularly combining alcohol with over-the-counter pain relievers, including acetaminophen or non-steroidal anti-inflammatory drugs, may increase your risk for liver damage.

Using alcohol to help relieve your pain also can lead to dependence and addiction. If you regularly drink more than a moderate amount of alcohol, talk with your doctor about the safest and most successful way to limit alcohol.

What's moderate drinking?

For most men, moderate drinking is no more than two drinks a day. That equals two 12-ounce (360-mL) cans of beer, two 5-ounce (150-mL) glasses of wine or two 1-ounce (30-mL) shot glasses of 100-proof whiskey.

For women and small-framed men, moderate drinking is half that—no more than one drink daily. The amount is less because women and smaller-sized men generally absorb more alcohol.

Quitting smoking

There's no question smoking is dangerous to your health. Tobacco smoke contains more than 4,000 substances that can damage your heart and blood vessels and cause cancer. Smoking also contributes to chronic pain by increasing fatigue and muscle weakness. Carbon monoxide in tobacco smoke replaces oxygen in your red blood cells. Less oxygen means less energy and fewer nutrients to your body tissues.

Breaking tobacco's grip

Some people can simply stop and never smoke again. For others, quitting takes several tries and various approaches. Don't let one bad experience keep you from trying again. You can learn from previous attempts, increasing your chances for being successful in the future.

Following these steps can help you snuff out tobacco for good:

Step 1: Do your homework. That way you'll know what to expect. You may experience physical withdrawal symptoms for at least 10 days. Common symptoms include irritability, anxiety and loss of concentration. Afterward, you may still have the urge to light up in familiar smoking situations, such as after a meal or while driving. These urges are generally very brief, but they can be very strong.

By knowing what to expect and having alternative activities planned, you'll be better prepared to handle the urges. These activities might include chewing gum after a meal or snacking on some carrot sticks or pretzels while driving to keep your hands busy.

Step 2: Set a stop date. Quitting cold turkey seems to work better than cutting down gradually. Carefully select a date to quit smoking.

Many smokers choose to quit during vacation. One reason is that your routine changes on vacation. It's easier to break free of smoking rituals than when you're at work or home.

Step 3: Tell others about your decision. Having the support of family, friends and coworkers can help you reach your goal more quickly. However, many smokers keep their plans to quit a secret because they don't want to look like a failure if they go back to smoking. Many people try three or more times before they're successful.

Step 4: Start changing your routine. Before your stop date, cut down on the number of places you smoke. For instance, stop smoking in your car, and smoke in only one room of the house or outside.

Medications to help you quit

These medications can reduce the difficult side effects of nicotine withdrawal and make quitting smoking easier. Use them according to your doctor's instructions, gradually tapering their use over a period of weeks to months.

Nicotine patches. Available as over-the-counter products and by prescription, the nicotine patch is placed on your skin, where it gradually releases nicotine into your body. This helps reduce nicotine cravings when you cut back or stop smoking. The patches can irritate your skin, but you can minimize the irritation by rotating the site of the patch and applying an over-the-counter cortisone cream.

Nicotine gum. You can also purchase over-the-counter nicotine gum. Bite into it a few times, then "park" it between your cheek and gum. The lining of your mouth absorbs the nicotine the gum releases. Nicotine gum can satisfy your nicotine urge, the same as the patch.

Nicotine nasal spray. It helps you quit in the same way as the patch or gum, but instead you spray nicotine into your nose. There, it's quickly absorbed into your bloodstream through the lining of your nose, providing quicker response to nicotine cravings than the other products. It's intended mainly for when you need a quick "hit" of nicotine. The product is available only by prescription.

Nicotine inhaler. This medication is available only by prescription. The device looks like a plastic cigarette. One end of the inhaler has a plastic tip like that used on some cigars. When you put this tip in your mouth and inhale, like puffing on a cigarette, the inhaler releases a nicotine vapor into your mouth, reducing your craving for nicotine. It also helps smokers who miss smoking's hand-to-mouth ritual.

Non-nicotine medication. Bupropion (Wellbutrin, Zyban) is the first non-nicotine medication approved by the Food and Drug Administration as a stop-smoking aid. It mimics some of the action of nicotine by releasing the brain chemicals dopamine and norepinephrine. Bupropion is also available only by prescription.

This approach will help reduce your smoking urges so you can be more comfortable in those places without smoking.

Step 5: Talk with your doctor about medications. Nicotine is a highly addictive substance. Withdrawal from nicotine can cause irritability, anxiety and difficulty concentrating. Medications are available that can help lessen withdrawal symptoms and increase your chances of being successful (see "Medications to help you quit" on previous page).

Step 6: Take one day at a time. On your stop day, quit completely. Each day, focus your attention on remaining tobacco-free.

Step 7: Avoid smoking situations. Leave the table immediately after meals if this is the time you used to light up. Take a walk instead. If you smoked while using the telephone, avoid long phone conversations or change the place where you talk. If you had a favorite smoking chair, avoid it.

You'll soon be able to anticipate when the urge to smoke will hit you. Before it hits, start doing something that makes smoking inconvenient, such as washing your car or doing relaxation exercises. Your smoking behavior is deeply ingrained and automatic. You need to anticipate your reflex behavior and plan alternatives.

Step 8: Time each urge. Check your watch when a smoking urge hits. Most are short. Once you realize this, it's easier to resist. Tell yourself, "I can make it another few minutes and then the urge will pass."

Expressing your sexuality

Sexuality is a natural and healthy part of living, and a part of your identity as a man or woman. It involves the timeless desire for both physical and emotional intimacy.

Sexuality can be expressed through shared interests, companionship or holding hands. A more physical expression of sexuality is physical contact, including sexual intercourse.

When chronic pain invades your life, the pleasures of sexuality often disappear. You may not feel like socializing, sharing your thoughts and feelings or having close contact. Perhaps you feel your pain has made you less desirable to your partner. Your sleeping arrangement may even have changed. Some people sleep in a spare bedroom or a lounger because they have difficulty getting comfortable or they don't want to keep their partner awake.

In spite of your pain, you can have a healthy and satisfying sexual relationship. It begins with honest communication. You and your partner need to talk about how you feel, what you miss and what you want or need from your relationship. You also need to be creative and willing to make changes. That could be as basic as purchasing a new mattress or a bigger bed so you don't have to sleep apart, or exploring different ways to express your sexuality.

In all partnerships it takes effort to maintain what is good and to correct what isn't. A healthy sexual relationship can positively affect all aspects of your life, including your physical health, self-esteem, productivity and other relationships.

Becoming more intimate

Start slowly. Before concentrating on improving your sexual relationship, spend time talking. Get to know one another again. Also look for ways to rekindle your romance. Go on a date, plan a picnic, send flowers or exchange personal gifts.

Remind yourself that problems are also opportunities. In your efforts to become more intimate you may discover something about your partner you otherwise might have missed. The relationship you recover may be even better than the one you had before your pain.

Fears about resuming sexual intercourse

You or your partner may have unspoken fears regarding sexual contact and, because of this, may avoid intimate encounters. Delaying intimacy only increases the anxiety surrounding sexual intercourse. Talking openly with your partner about your fears can help ease them.

Fear of increased pain. It's natural to want to avoid additional pain. And it's common to worry that sexual intercourse will cause you physical pain, especially if your pain is centered in your back, abdomen or pelvis.

Experimenting with different positions and other ways to satisfy your and your partner's sexual needs can help the two of you enjoy intimate encounters (see "Making love creatively" on following page). Remember, sexuality is not just the act of sexual intercourse. It's any action that connects you intimately with another person.

Fear of partner rejection. This is a common feeling. You may wonder if your partner is less attracted to you because of your pain. The longer you have these fears, the more difficult it may be to overcome them.

Making love creatively

Sexual intercourse is just one way to satisfy your need for human closeness. Intimacy can be expressed in many different ways.

Touch. Exploring your partner's body through touch is an exciting way to express your sexual feelings. This can include cuddling, fondling, stroking, massaging and kissing. Touch in any form increases feelings of intimacy.

Self-stimulation. Masturbation is a normal and healthy way to fulfill your sexual needs. One partner may use masturbation during mutual sexual activity if the other partner is unable to be very active.

Oral sex. It can be an alternative or supplement to traditional intercourse.

Timing and positions. A change in the time of day you have sexual intercourse may improve your lovemaking. Many people often have higher pain levels in the evening. If this is true for you, you and your partner might try intercourse in the morning or afternoon.

Experiment with different positions. Lay side by side, kneel or sit. There are many good books in bookstores and medical libraries that describe different ways to have intercourse.

Vibrators and lubricants. A vibrator can add pleasure without physical exertion. If lack of natural lubrication is a problem, over-the-counter lubricants can prevent pain associated with vaginal dryness.

Talk openly with your partner about your feelings and fears and encourage your partner to do the same.

Fear of failure to perform. If you're having difficulty becoming sexually aroused, maintaining an erection or achieving an orgasm, talk with your doctor. Your pain itself, depression, concern over your physical appearance, alcohol and medications can all affect your sexual performance.

Antidepressants and sedatives are some of the drugs that can reduce your sexual ability, including making you impotent. If you suspect a medication may be affecting your sexual performance, don't stop taking the drug without first consulting your doctor.

Sometimes, failure to perform is simply a result of stress and anxiety. Patience and understanding can often help you overcome the problem.

Addressing your spiritual needs

Spirituality is an important aspect of well-being that many people tend to overlook.

Spirituality is often confused with religion. But spirituality isn't so much connected to a specific belief or form of worship as it is with the spirit or the soul. Spirituality is about meaning, values and purpose in life.

Religion may be one way of expressing spirituality, but it's not the only way. For some people, spirituality is feeling in tune with nature and the universe. For still others, spirituality is expressed through music, meditation or art.

Addressing your spiritual needs can be an effective strategy for managing chronic pain. People find it brings inner peace and added strength to deal with their pain and stress.

Spirituality and healing

Numerous studies have attempted to measure the effect of spirituality on illness and recovery. In reviewing many of these studies, researchers at Georgetown University School of Medicine found that at least 80 percent of the studies suggested spiritual beliefs have a beneficial effect on health. The researchers concluded that people who consider themselves to be spiritual enjoy better health, live longer, recover from illness more quickly and with fewer complications, suffer less depression and chemical addiction, have lower blood pressure and cope better with serious disease, such as cancer and cardiovascular disease.

No one knows exactly how spirituality affects health. Some experts attribute the healing effect to hope, which is known to benefit your immune system. Others liken spiritual acts and beliefs to meditation, which decreases muscle tension and can lower your heart rate. Still others point to the social connectedness spirituality often provides.

An important point to keep in mind: Although spirituality is associated with healing and better health, it isn't a cure. Spirituality can help you live life more fully despite your symptoms, but studies haven't found that it actually cures health problems. It's best to view spirituality as a helpful healing force, but not a substitute for traditional medical care.

Finding spiritual well-being

The first step toward reclaiming a sense of spiritual well-being is to recognize what actions, feelings, people or circumstances are interfering with your sense of inner peace. Once you recognize what is making you angry, anxious, nervous or stressed, you can begin to respond effectively.

Use the coping and problem-solving skills discussed in Chapter 9 (page 90) to help you deal with the emotions or circumstances that are troubling you. If you decide that whatever is making you angry, anxious, nervous or stressed is beyond your control, you need to recognize this and "let go."

Many people find that talking openly with a therapist, religious leader or their doctor helps them find internal peace. Other methods of gaining inner peace include relaxation techniques, inspirational writings, worship, prayer, volunteer work, art, music and spending time in the outdoors.

Chapter 12

What About Medication?

For acute pain, medication is often the first line of treatment. And usually it's effective. After a while, the pain diminishes or disappears.

With chronic pain, the solution usually isn't that simple. Unlike acute pain, which generally responds well to medication, medications aren't always effective for chronic pain. Long-term use of pain medications also can cause side effects, including stomach-related problems, liver damage and dependency. And, sometimes, medication can actually make your pain worse.

However, that doesn't mean medication may never be part of your treatment. Medications can sometimes effectively reduce chronic pain with limited side effects. They can also help control a temporary flare in your pain. In addition, medications can help treat other conditions that may accompany chronic pain, such as depression or difficulty sleeping.

This chapter looks at various medications and drug-related therapies to help you understand why some medications and therapies may be OK, why you should limit others and why it may be best to avoid all medication.

Simple pain relievers

Pain medications, called analgesics (AN-ul-JE-siks), are the most widely used medication. They control pain in various ways—by interfering with the development of pain messages, their frequency, path or interpretation.

Here are the most common over-the-counter and prescription pain relievers.

Nonsteroidal anti-inflammatory drugs (NSAIDs)

NSAIDs (en-SAYDS) are most effective for mild to moderate pain accompanied by swelling and inflammation. The drugs relieve pain by inhibiting an enzyme in your body called cyclooxygenase (SI-klo-OX-suh-juhn-ays). This enzyme makes hormonelike substances called prostaglandins involved in the development of pain and inflammation.

NSAIDs are especially helpful for arthritis and pain resulting from muscle sprains, strains, back and neck injuries or cramps.

Over-the-counter NSAIDs include:
- aspirin (Bayer, Excedrin and others)
- ibuprofen (Advil, Motrin IB, Nuprin)
- ketoprofen (Actron, Orudis KT)
- naproxen sodium (Aleve)

NSAIDs available only by prescription include:
- diclofenac sodium (Voltaren XR)
- etodolac (Lodine XL)
- fenoprofen (Nalfon)
- flurbiprofen (Ansaid)
- indomethacin (Indocin)
- ketorolac tromethamine (Toradol)
- nabumetone (Relafen)
- naproxen (Anaprox DS, Naprelan, Naprosyn)
- oxaprozin (Daypro)
- piroxicam (Feldene)
- sulindac (Clinoril)

When taken occasionally and as directed, NSAIDs are generally safe. But if you take them regularly for months to years, or if you take more than the recommended dosage, NSAIDs may cause nausea, stomach pain, stomach bleeding or ulcers. Large doses of NSAIDs also can lead to kidney problems, fluid retention and heart failure. Risk for these conditions increases with age, especially among women. If you regularly take NSAIDs, talk to your doctor so he or she can monitor for side effects.

NSAIDs also have a "ceiling effect." There's a limit as to how much pain the drugs can control. Beyond a certain dosage they don't provide any additional benefit. If you have moderate to severe pain, that limit may not be enough to relieve your pain adequately.

Cox-2 inhibitors

These are newer NSAIDs that appear to be less damaging to your stomach. They include the prescription drugs:
- celecoxib (Celebrex)
- rofecoxib (Vioxx)

Cyclooxygenase comes in two forms, called cox-1 and cox-2. Unlike other NSAIDs, cox-2 inhibitors suppress only one form of cyclooxygenase. Researchers believe part of the role of cox-1 is to protect your stomach lining. When NSAIDs suppress its function, side effects such as stomach, intestinal and kidney problems can result.

Cox-2 inhibitors affect only that form of the enzyme (cox-2) involved in inflammation. Because they don't affect cox-1, the drugs don't appear to be as harmful to your digestive system.

In studies of cox-2 inhibitors, participants reported a 30 percent to 70 percent reduction in pain without common side effects associated with traditional NSAIDs. However, long-term effects of cox-2 inhibitors are unknown.

Acetaminophen

Acetaminophen is most effective for minor to moderate pain that isn't accompanied by inflammation. Unlike cox-2 inhibitors and other NSAIDs, acetaminophen doesn't affect prostaglandins. Therefore, it does little to reduce inflammation.

Over-the-counter brands of acetaminophen include:
- Anacin-3
- Aspirin-Free Anacin
- Aspirin-Free Excedrin
- Panadol
- Tylenol

When taken occasionally and as recommended, acetaminophen is safe. However, if you frequently take more of the drug than recommended on the product label, it could possibly lead to liver damage. Alcohol appears to enhance the risk. If you regularly combine too much acetaminophen with alcohol, your chances for liver damage are increased.

Acetaminophen is sometimes combined with a narcotic to provide stronger pain relief. This form of the drug is available only by prescription. Taken regularly, it can become habit-forming.

As with NSAIDs, if you frequently take acetaminophen, make sure your doctor is aware so he or she can monitor for possible side effects.

Ointments

These drugs come in the form of a cream or a gel. Instead of breaking down in your digestive tract and moving through your central nervous system, they're absorbed through your skin.

Pain-relief ointments can occasionally help relieve nerve pain and inflammation just below your skin. Three types of ointments are available over-the-counter:

Capsaicin. This drug is made from the seeds of hot chili peppers. It works by depleting your nerve cells of a chemical called substance P involved in transmitting pain messages.

You periodically rub capsaicin (Capzasin-P, Dolorac and Zostrix) on your skin, typically three or four times a day. It usually takes about 1 to 2 weeks before you begin to feel noticeable pain relief. If you miss one or two applications, it will take longer for the drug to work.

Capsaicin is most effective for arthritic joints close to your skin surface, such as your fingers, knees and elbows. It may also help relieve pain after shingles (postherpetic neuralgia), pain from diabetes (diabetic neuropathy) and chronic pain near healed surgical scars.

Because the drug is generally safe and effective, you can use it long-term. However, it can temporarily irritate your skin and produce a burning sensation.

Methyl products. These medications (ArthriCare, Ben-Gay, and Icy Hot) use heat or cold to cover up, or "counter," the existing pain.

Methyl-related products may relieve occasional, mild muscle aches, but they're not effective for most forms of chronic pain. In addition, they typically require frequent applications, and some products have a medicinal smell.

Aspirin products. Medications such as Aspercreme, Sportscreme and Myoflex contain trolamine salicylate (TRO-lah-MEEN SAL-i-sil-AYT), a chemical that's similar to aspirin. The Food and Drug Administration lists these drugs as safe, but not necessarily effective for pain relief.

Potent painkillers

These prescription medications are taken most often to relieve pain from cancer, a terminal illness, severe injury or surgery. Pain control after surgery is especially important because the sooner you're active, the less risk for complications, such as pneumonia or blood clots, due to inactivity.

Narcotics

Some narcotics are natural compounds derived from opium. Others are synthetic medications that work in a similar fashion.

Narcotics include:

- butorphanol (Stadol)
- codeine (aspirin with codeine, Tylenol with codeine)
- fentanyl (Duragesic, Sublimaze)
- hydrocodone (Lorcet, Lortab, Vicodin and others)
- hydromorphone (Dilaudid)
- levorphanol (Levo-Dromoran)
- meperidine (Demerol)
- methadone (Dolophine)
- morphine (Duramorph, MS Contin, Roxanol and others)
- oxycodone (Percocet, Roxicet, Tylox and others)
- oxymorphone (Numorphan)
- propoxyphene (Darvon, Darvocet)

When taken for short periods, narcotics generally cause only minor side effects, such as nausea, constipation, sedation and unclear thinking. But when taken for several weeks to months, these side effects can become more bothersome. The drugs also can lose their effectiveness as your body develops a tolerance to the drug.

When drugs worsen the pain

If you take a pain medication regularly, sometimes the drug can make your pain worse instead of better. This is called rebound pain.

Although scientists don't know for certain what causes rebound pain, they think that overuse of pain medication may somehow short-circuit your brain's pain control systems. When your medication wears off, your pain returns with a vengeance. To deal with the pain, you take more medication. This results in an unending cycle of severe pain and increased drug use.

Virtually any pain reliever can cause rebound pain. The best way to deal with this problem is to gradually wean yourself from your medication with help from your doctor. Your pain may worsen for a few days, then gradually improve.

Arguably, though, the biggest concern with narcotics is risk of physical dependence or addiction (see page 40). Narcotics can become habit-forming, and that's why doctors have generally limited their use to acute pain. In recent years, however, there's been some difference of opinion regarding these drugs. More doctors have begun prescribing narcotics for chronic pain in response to studies that suggest the risk of addiction is less than once thought.

Several studies show that most people who regularly take a narcotic become physically dependent on the drug and experience some minor withdrawal symptoms if they stop using it abruptly. But only a small percentage of people actually abuse the drug or become psychologically addicted to it. Although addiction is a serious problem, physical dependence itself may not result in serious problems, provided the medication is being taken as directed.

Still, many doctors believe the side effects and potential risks associated with long-term use of narcotics for chronic pain remain too high to justify their use. Plus, it isn't always possible to determine who may be at high risk for addiction.

Tramadol

Tramadol (Ultram) is a prescription pain medication that works in two ways. Like a narcotic, it interferes with the transmission of pain signals.

A steady stream of relief

For some people with excruciating pain that isn't helped by other measures, one option to control the pain is a pain pump. The small device is surgically implanted in your lower abdomen, where it provides a steady injection of medication—typically a narcotic—to your spinal cord. Sometimes a combination of drugs, such as a narcotic combined with a muscle relaxant and local anesthetic, is included.

Pain pumps are used most often to control pain associated with a terminal illness or severe nerve damage. Because surgery carries risks and narcotics can cause serious side effects, the devices are generally a last resort when other methods haven't worked. Most people who receive a pain pump continue to experience pain, but the pump dulls the pain enough to make it tolerable.

The drug also triggers release of the brain hormones norepinephrine and serotonin that help reduce pain.

Tramadol is used mainly to relieve moderate to severe acute pain. Its use in chronic pain hasn't been well studied. In a few studies where the drug was prescribed for chronic pain, some people experienced significant pain relief, but others had no relief at all.

Because it's a weak narcotic, risk for physical dependence and addiction is low. Side effects from tramadol can include dizziness, sedation, headache, nausea and constipation. Possible long-term effects from the drug are unknown.

Other pain medications

Ironically, some of the more effective and commonly used medications for chronic pain are drugs that were developed to control other conditions. Following are medications that typically don't fall under the heading of analgesics but can also reduce pain.

Tricyclic antidepressants
In addition to relieving symptoms of depression, these drugs interfere with certain chemical processes in your brain that cause you to feel pain. They include:
- amitriptyline (Elavil, Endep)
- amoxapine (Asendin)
- clomipramine (Anafranil)
- desipramine (Norpramin)
- doxepin (Sinequan)
- imipramine (Tofranil)
- nortriptyline (Aventyl, Pamelor)
- protriptyline (Vivactil)
- trimipramine (Surmontil)

Unlike narcotics, antidepressants don't cause dependency or addiction. However, tricyclic antidepressants can make you drowsy. Therefore, it's generally recommended that you take the medication in the evening before bed. In addition, the drugs may cause dry mouth, constipation, difficulty with urination and weight gain. To reduce or prevent these symptoms, your doctor will likely start you off at a low dose and slowly increase the amount of the drug you take. Most people are able to take tricyclic antidepressants with only mild side effects.

Anti-seizure medications

Developed primarily to reduce or control epileptic seizures, these medications also help control stabbing, shooting or jabbing pain from nerve damage. The drugs seem to work by quieting damaged nerves to slow or prevent them from sending uncontrolled pain signals.

Anti-seizure medications used for chronic pain include:

- carbamazepine (Carbatrol, Tegretol)
- gabapentin (Neurontin)
- lamotrigine (Lamictal)
- phenytoin (Dilantin)

These medications can cause dizziness, drowsiness, nausea and constipation. But, again, most people are bothered only minimally. More severe but less common side effects include blood, heart and liver disorders. To reduce your risk for side effects, your doctor will likely start you off on a small amount of the drug and gradually increase the dose over a period of several weeks.

Medications for associated conditions

Relief from your pain isn't the only reason you may take medication. Drugs may not reduce your pain, but they can relieve other troubling symptoms associated with chronic pain. This is important because when you aren't affected by other symptoms, you can direct more of your energy toward your daily activities.

Depression

Relief from depression can have a significant effect on your ability to manage your pain. As you begin to feel better and more energetic, your pain seems more tolerable.

Experts believe depression may result from an imbalance in certain brain chemicals (neurotransmitters) that affect your mood and emotions. The condition is often treated with medications that increase production of these chemicals. In addition to tricyclic antidepressants, discussed earlier, other types of antidepressants include:

Selective serotonin reuptake inhibitors (SSRIs). These medications have become the first-line treatment for depression because they produce few serious side effects. The drugs seem to work by increasing the availability of the neurotransmitter serotonin.

Medications to control migraines

If your migraines don't respond to common pain medications, your doctor may recommend one or more of these drugs:

Preventive drugs

Medications to prevent or reduce migraines:

Cardiovascular drugs. This includes beta blockers and calcium channel blockers. How they control migraines is unclear.

Antidepressants. Tricyclic antidepressants increase levels of the hormone serotonin and other brain chemicals.

Anti-seizure drugs. Valproic acid (Depakote) is the drug most commonly used. Its mechanism of action also is uncertain.

Serotonin antagonists. Drugs such as cyproheptadine (Periactin) and methysergide (Sansert) diminish the effects of serotonin.

Riboflavin (vitamin B_2). A riboflavin deficiency may contribute to recurring headaches. High doses of vitamin B_2 (400 milligrams per day) can correct the deficiency. Take high doses of this vitamin only with medical supervision.

Abortive drugs

Drugs that help relieve migraine symptoms:

Sumatriptan. It mimics the brain chemical serotonin, deactivating nerves and shrinking swollen blood vessels. Sumatriptan (Imitrex) comes in pill, injection or nasal spray form. Similar drugs include naratriptan (Amerge), rizatriptan (Maxalt) and zolmitriptan (Zomig).

Vasoconstrictors. The drugs dihydroergotamine (D.H.E. 45) and ergotamine (Ercaf, Ergomar, Wigraine) influence brain hormone receptors, including serotonin receptors.

Mixed analgesics. They include Fioricet, Fiorinal and Midrin, which contain a combination of medications, including acetaminophen.

Lidocaine nasal drops. They contain an anesthetic that works on nasal passage nerves. The drops often relieve pain within a few minutes, but in about 40 percent of people the pain returns.

SSRIs include the prescription medications:
- citalopram (Celexa)
- fluoxetine (Prozac)
- fluvoxamine (Luvox)
- paroxetine (Paxil)
- sertraline (Zoloft)

SSRIs, however, can cause sexual problems in up to 30 percent of people. Once you stop taking the drug, the problems usually disappear.

Other antidepressants that work similar to SSRIs but affect different neurotransmitters include:
- bupropion (Wellbutrin)
- maprotiline (Ludiomil)
- mirtazapine (Remeron)
- nefazodone (Serzone)
- trazodone (Desyrel)
- venlafaxine (Effexor)

Monoamine oxidase inhibitors. These drugs are generally prescribed only if other antidepressants aren't effective. They include:
- phenelzine (Nardil)
- tranylcypromine (Parnate)

The drugs can interact with certain foods and other medications to cause serious side effects, including an increase in your blood pressure and heart rate, chest pain and trouble breathing. Less serious and more common side effects include feeling light-headed or dizzy.

Lithium and mood-stabilizing medications. This group of drugs is used to treat bipolar disorder (manic-depressive illness), which involves recurrent cycles of emotions at both extremes, elation and depression.

It includes these medications:
- carbamazepine (Epitol, Tegretol)
- gabapentin (Neurontin)
- lithium (Eskalith, Lithobid)
- valproate (Depakene, Depakote)

Sleep loss

A good night's sleep can help you better cope with your pain by renewing your energy level and improving your mood. Medications that promote sleep include:

Antidepressants. Drowsiness is a common side effect of some antidepressants. When taken at night before bed, the drugs may help you sleep better—in addition to controlling pain and depression.

Sedatives. These medications help promote sleep. However, they can cloud your thinking, make you drowsy, impair your balance and affect your ability to drive. If taken regularly, they may also cause dependency or addiction.

Prescription sedatives include:

- alprazolam (Xanax)
- butabarbital sodium (Butisol Sodium)
- chlordiazepoxide (Librium)
- clonazepam (Klonopin)
- clorazepate (Tranxene)
- diazepam (Valium)
- estazolam (ProSom)
- flurazepam (Dalmane)
- lorazepam (Ativan)
- oxazepam (Serax)
- pentobarbital sodium (Nembutal Sodium)
- triazolam (Halcion)
- zolpidem (Ambien)

Zolpidem is a newer type of sleep medication that causes more natural sleep and isn't as likely to lead to addiction as other sedatives.

Muscle spasms

If your pain is accompanied by muscle spasms, your doctor may recommend a muscle relaxant to control the spasms. However, take these drugs only occasionally. When taken regularly, they can cloud your thinking and leave you drowsy and dizzy.

Muscle relaxants include the prescription drugs:

- baclofen (Lioresal)
- carisoprodol (Soma)
- chlorzoxazone (Parafon Forte)
- cyclobenzaprine (Flexeril)
- methocarbamol (Robaxin)
- orphenadrine (Norflex)

For more on medications, visit MayoClinic.com

If you want to learn more about a drug you're taking, visit our Web site at *www.MayoClinic.com*.

Injections

Sometimes, instead of taking pills to control your pain, a more effective approach is to inject medication at or near the pain site. Injections are most effective for nerve, joint or muscle pain confined to a specific location. They may include an anesthetic to control the pain, a steroid to reduce inflammation or a combination of the two.

The benefit of injections is that the medication works primarily on the injected area. However, your doctor needs to administer the injections, and their effects often are only temporary. In addition, there's a limit as to how often you can receive an injection, depending on the location where it's given and the medication used. Overuse of steroids can lead to a number of side effects, including loss of bone mass, muscle weakness, accumulation of fat around your face and increased risk for cataracts.

Injections typically aren't a cure, but they can help some people through an initial period of intense pain or a severe flare in their pain.

Nerve blocks

A nerve block involves injecting an anesthetic around a nerve's fibers, preventing pain messages traveling along that nerve pathway from reaching your brain. Nerve blocks are used most often to relieve pain for a short period until other therapies or medications can take effect. Depending on how well you respond to the injection, a nerve block can reduce pain for a few days to several months.

There are three main types of nerve blocks:

Peripheral. An anesthetic is injected at a specific location, such as an ankle, to reduce feeling and pain in that localized area.

Spinal. For pain that affects a broader area, such as your lower back or a leg, an anesthetic is injected near a major nerve at the base of your spine to reduce pain all the way down the path of the nerve to your toes.

Sympathetic. Some forms of chronic pain, such as complex regional pain syndrome, may result from abnormal activity of your sympathetic nervous system. Your sympathetic nerves control circulation and per-spiration and are part of your automatic nervous system. To prevent messages produced by your sympathetic nerves from reaching your brain, an anesthetic may be injected near the painful area or on the sympathetic nerve.

Trigger-point injections

With this type of injection, medication is directed into a muscle, rather

Self-care for pain control

For mild to moderate muscle and joint pain, cold and heat can often be as effective as medication, without the risks and costs.

Cold

Ice decreases pain by numbing the area. It works best for muscle spasms or swelling and joint pain.

Ice massage. Rub a block of ice over the area for 5 to 7 minutes until it becomes slightly numb. Watch for color changes in your skin. If you notice your skin losing its underlying red tone, stop immediately. It could indicate the onset of frostbite. If your skin becomes numb during the massage, end the treatment early.

Cold packs. Place a damp towel over the painful area. Put the cold pack on the towel and cover it with dry towels for insulation. Don't leave the pack on the area for more than 20 minutes at a time. Check your skin regularly for loss of underlying redness.

Heat

Heat increases blood flow and nutrients to painful muscles and joints. It also helps improve flexibility.

Hot packs. Place several towels over the painful area. Lay the hot pack on top. Cover the pack with more towels for insulation. Add or remove towels between your skin and the pack to vary the heat. Check your skin every 15 minutes. If you see red and white blotches, stop the treatment at once to prevent a burn.

Heating pads. Place a towel over the painful area and put the pad on top. Limit use of a heating pad to 30 minutes at a time. Check occasionally for red and white blotches.

Heat lamps. Use a 250-watt reflector heat bulb. It produces infrared rays that increase blood circulation. Position the lamp 18 to 20 inches from your skin. To decrease the heat intensity, move the lamp farther away. Apply heat to the sore area for no longer than 30 minutes. If you think you might fall asleep, use an alarm clock or timer.

Baths and hot tubs. A 15-minute hot bath can be just as effective as a hot tub. Don't get the water too hot so that you burn yourself. If you have a hot tub, limit its use to no more than 30 minutes a time.

than around a nerve. Depending on the medication used, trigger-point injections can reduce pain in the muscle, reduce inflammation or relax a muscle that's producing spasms. An acute flare of pain or swelling is the most common reason for these injections.

The medication crutch

Medication may seem like an easy way to control your pain, but it's often not the best way. Even pain medications that are considered safe can cause side effects. Medications also can become a crutch. People take them because they feel they need to, not because the drugs are helping. These people are often surprised to find that withdrawal from their medication isn't as difficult as they anticipated. They also find that life without drugs gives them a greater sense of control over their pain and life.

If you take pain medication regularly, including over-the-counter products, discuss your medication, its benefits and its side effects with your doctor. You should know the type of medication you're taking, why you're taking it and possible effects from the drug. You may be attributing your fatigue, stomach discomfort or sexual problems to your pain, when it's really your medication that's causing these symptoms.

If you take a narcotic or another habit-forming drug, ask your doctor if it would be in your best interest to taper use of the drug. Before you begin your drug withdrawal, ask about side effects you may experience, such as anxiety and nausea, and discuss ways to lessen these effects. Your doctor will probably want to see you regularly during this period to measure your vital signs and make sure the withdrawal doesn't trigger other health problems.

Depending on the severity of your pain and the type of medication you're taking, your initial goal may be simply to change to a safer medication or reduce the amount of medication you take. However, as you become more comfortable in your role as pain manager, you may want to consider eliminating your use of all pain medications and rely on other methods to manage your pain, including changes in your lifestyle, and use of cold and heat.

Some people need medication to treat a specific condition. But you may be among those who can control your pain as, or more, effectively without drugs.

Chapter 13

Complementary and Alternative Medicine

*I*n your effort to find relief from your pain, chances are you've tried, or at least considered, some form of complementary or alternative medicine. Maybe you've had a massage, practiced meditation or yoga or thought about acupuncture or herbal medicines.

And you probably have a lot of questions. Do these methods really work? Are they safe? Exactly what is complementary and alternative medicine?

Complementary and alternative medicine cover a broad range of healing philosophies, approaches and therapies that aren't widely taught in medical schools, used in hospitals or reimbursed by health insurance companies. Although the two terms are often used synonymously, they aren't the same.

The National Center for Complementary and Alternative Medicine, a division of the National Institutes of Health, defines alternative medicine as therapies or healing approaches used by themselves, in place of traditional medicine. This might include seeing a homeopathic or naturopathic practitioner for your medical care. Complementary medicine refers to unconventional medical practices used in addition to the treatments recommended by your doctor: for example, incorporating biofeedback and Tai Chi with diet and exercise.

Alternative and complementary therapies aren't new. Some have been practiced for thousands of years. But their use has become more popular as Americans seek greater control of their own health. Two of the most common reasons people use alternative and complementary medicine are for treatment of anxiety and pain.

Does that mean they work? Several treatments do appear to safely relieve stress and reduce pain, and gradually, many of these therapies are gaining acceptance within mainstream medicine. But there are many products and practices that remain unproven because they haven't been adequately studied.

Here's a look at some of the more common complementary and alternative treatments promoted for pain management.

The mind and body connection

These practices are based on the interconnectedness of mind and body, and the power of one to affect the other. They've been shown to help control chronic pain by reducing stress, tension and depression, factors that intensify pain. Mind and body therapies also help promote an overall sense of well-being.

Biofeedback

This practice uses technology to teach you how to control certain body responses that help reduce pain. During a biofeedback session, a trained therapist applies electrodes and other sensors to various parts of your body. The electrodes are attached to devices that monitor and give you feedback on bodily functions, including muscle tension, brain wave activity, heart rate, blood pressure and temperature.

Once the electrodes are in place, the therapist uses relaxation techniques to calm you, reducing muscle tension and slowing your heart rate and breathing. You then learn how to produce these changes yourself. The goal of biofeedback is to help you enter a relaxed state in which you can better cope with your pain.

Biofeedback techniques are often taught in physical therapy or behavioral medicine departments in medical centers and hospitals.

Humor therapy

Humor therapy is based on the belief that regular periods of laughter help distract your attention from your pain. Laughter is also a type of analgesic. It promotes the release of chemicals that block pain messages. By this action, laughter helps reduce pain.

Humor therapy involves spending a few minutes each day laughing. You might watch a funny movie, call a friend who makes you laugh, joke with your neighbors or coworkers or visit a comedy club.

Humor therapy also may help increase muscle flexibility and lower blood pressure.

Hypnosis

People have been using hypnosis to promote healing since ancient times. However, in the past 50 years, it's experienced a resurgence among physicians, psychologists and mental health professionals.

Hypnosis produces an induced state of relaxation in which your mind stays narrowly focused and open to suggestion. No one knows how hypnosis works, but experts believe it alters your brain-wave patterns in much the same way as other relaxation techniques.

For treatment of chronic pain, you receive suggestions designed to help you decrease your perception of the pain and increase your ability to cope with it. Unlike situations sometimes portrayed in movies and on TV, you can't be forced under hypnosis to do something you normally wouldn't want to do.

The success of hypnosis depends on your understanding of the procedure and your willingness to try it. You need to be strongly motivated to change. About 80 percent of adults can be hypnotized by a trained professional. People who don't want to feel out of control often can't be. Psychiatrists and psychologists occasionally practice hypnosis. You can also undergo hypnosis from a professional hypnotist. Some people eventually develop the skills to hypnotize themselves. Once you're trained in self-hypnosis, you can use this technique, as needed, to manage your pain.

Meditation

Meditation is a way to calm your mind and body. It originates from various religious and cultural traditions.

During meditation you sit quietly and focus on nothing or on a "mantra"—a simple sound repeated over and over. This causes you to enter a deeply restful state that reduces your body's stress response. Your breathing slows, your muscles relax and your brain wave activity indicates a state of relaxation.

Regular meditation can help reduce anxiety and chronic pain. It may also reduce blood pressure and possibly even increase longevity.

Although meditation sounds simple, learning to control your thoughts isn't as easy as it may seem. The more you practice, though, the less difficult it becomes to hold your concentration without having your mind wander.

You can learn meditation from a trained instructor or from a psychiatrist or other mental health professional. Sometimes, meditation is used in conjunction with biofeedback to help promote relaxation.

Music, dance and art therapy

These therapies reduce stress and anxiety. They also help promote self-confidence and personal well-being, and may reduce symptoms of depression.

Like other forms of relaxation, graceful dance, art expression and performing or listening to music help reduce pain by relieving muscle tension and slowing your breathing.

Several national organizations promote the use of music, dance and art for health and healing. These organizations have chapters set up across the country (see pages 167 and 168 for details). In addition, some medical centers offer music, dance or art therapy programs.

Yoga

Yoga is a 5,000-year-old practice that incorporates proper breathing, movement and posture to achieve a union of mind, body and spirit. It involves completing a series of postures, during which you pay special attention to your breathing—exhaling during certain movements and inhaling with others.

A sizeable amount of research on yoga shows it can help control pain by relieving stress and anxiety. It also reduces your heart rate and slows your breathing. Studies show it has even helped some people stop smoking.

To be effective, yoga requires training and regular practice. You can find qualified instructors at yoga schools. You also can learn about yoga through books and videotapes. Depending on your type of pain, you may need to modify or avoid some of the yoga postures to prevent excessive stress to your muscles and joints.

Healing through manipulation and touch

These therapies and practices are designed to promote healing and relieve pain by manipulating body tissues. They're based on the belief that when one part of your body isn't functioning properly, other areas are affected.

Aromatherapy

This ancient form of healing uses essential oils derived from plant extracts and resins to promote both health and beauty. Practitioners believe these oils can help treat various conditions, including chronic pain, when massaged into your skin or inhaled.

At least 40 oils are used in aromatherapy, categorized according to their effects on mind, body and specific diseases.

Medical experts acknowledge that therapeutic massage may help reduce pain and muscle stiffness and promote relaxation. However, more study is needed to determine whether the oils used in aromatherapy provide any health benefit.

Chiropractic

Chiropractic medicine is perhaps the most commonly used alternative therapy in the United States. It's based on the belief that certain illnesses and conditions, including chronic pain, result from impairment of your nervous system, due to problems with your joints. To relieve or eliminate negative effects on your nerves, chiropractors manipulate associated joints, typically by slightly stretching or "adjusting" them.

There are two types of chiropractors. Those who depend solely on traditional chiropractic practices are referred to as "straight" practitioners. Chiropractors who combine standard chiropractic techniques with other therapies, such as exercise, acupuncture or dietary and herbal supplements, are known as "mixers."

The effectiveness of chiropractic therapies is controversial. Back pain is the most common reason people see a chiropractor, and studies indicate that for some types of low back pain, especially acute pain, chiropractic may be effective.

Massage

Massage therapy is one of the oldest methods of health care still in practice. It involves use of different manipulative techniques to move your body's muscles and soft tissues. A massage therapist primarily uses his or her hands to manipulate muscles and tissues, but sometimes a therapist may use his or her forearms, elbows or feet.

Massage therapy is based on the belief that when muscles are overworked, waste products can accumulate in the muscle, causing soreness and stiffness. The therapy aims to improve circulation in the muscle, increasing flow of nutrients and eliminating waste products.

Massage can reduce your heart rate, relax your muscles, improve range of motion in your joints and increase production of your body's natural painkillers. It often helps relieve stress and anxiety. It also can help relieve headaches and lower blood pressure. Although massage is almost always safe, avoid it if you have open sores, acute inflammation or circulatory problems.

"Movement" therapies

Several nontraditional therapies, such as the Feldenkrais and Trager methods, center around the philosophy that, over time, people start moving and holding their bodies in dysfunctional ways. Weaker muscles end up doing the work of stronger muscles, causing stress and tension.

An instructor takes you through a series of specific movements designed to teach you to use your muscles and joints more comfortably and efficiently. The movements also help you find greater pleasure in, and ease with, your body.

Practitioners claim these therapies can help control pain and promote an overall sense of well-being. Although they appear to be safe, their benefits aren't scientifically proven.

Osteopathy

Osteopathy is a recognized medical discipline that has much in common with conventional medicine. Similar to traditional physicians, doctors of osteopathy go through rigorous and lengthy training in academic and clinical settings. They're licensed to perform many of the same therapies and procedures as traditional doctors, including surgery and prescribing medications. They also may specialize in various forms of medicine, from gynecology to cardiology.

One area where osteopathy differs from conventional medicine is its reliance on manipulation to address joint and spinal problems. Similar in this respect to a chiropractor, an osteopath performs manipulations to try to release pressure in your joints and align your musculoskeletal structure to improve movement and flow of bodily fluids. However, some osteopaths don't rely as heavily on manipulation as others.

As with chiropractic medicine, the effectiveness of manipulation in improving mobility and relieving pain is controversial. However, many studies support osteopathic techniques for many joint- and muscle-related conditions.

Rolfing

This therapy uses deep massage to align your body so that all of its components are positioned correctly.

The theory behind Rolfing is that injury or stress causes tissues to adhere in unhealthful ways, interfering with your body's natural movement and producing symptoms such as fatigue and pain. To restore natural alignment, a "Rolfer" applies deep pressure in an attempt to stretch the tissues and help reposition your muscles and joints.

There are no scientific studies to prove Rolfing's benefits. Its deep massage may help reduce stress and tension. However, some people find the procedure painful.

Restoring natural energy forces

Several complementary and alternative medicines are based on the belief that internal and external energy forces play a role in health and healing. Studies show some of these therapies may help reduce chronic pain. For others, there's little, if any, evidence to prove their benefits.

Acupressure

Acupressure, like acupuncture, stems from the Chinese belief that just below your skin are 14 invisible pathways, called meridians. Through these pathways flow chi (CHEE), the Chinese word for "life force." When the flow of chi is interrupted, illness results.

During acupressure, a practitioner applies pressure with his or her finger to specific points on your body to restore free flow of chi and relieve symptoms such as pain and stress.

Research on the benefits of acupressure is inconclusive. Many people who feel they're helped by the procedure find its hands-on therapy to be relaxing and comforting.

Acupuncture

Acupuncture is one of the most studied unconventional medical practices, and it's slowly gaining acceptance into Westernized medicine for treatment of certain conditions. A consensus statement on acupuncture released in 1998 by the National Institutes of Health states there's enough evidence to prove that acupuncture helps relieve postoperative dental pain and nausea caused by chemotherapy, anesthesia or pregnancy.

The report also concludes that acupuncture may help control pain associated with low-back problems, migraines, osteoarthritis, fibromyalgia and carpal tunnel syndrome.

During a typical acupuncture session, an acupuncturist inserts anywhere from 1 to 10 hair-thin needles into your skin for 15 to 40 minutes. The purpose of the needles is to remove blockages in the meridians and promote the free flow of chi. The acupuncturist may also manipulate the needles or apply electrical stimulation or heat to the needles. There should be little or no pain from insertion of the needles. Some people even find the procedure relaxing.

Adverse side effects from acupuncture are rare, but they can occur. Make sure your acupuncturist is trained and follows good hygiene practices, including use of disposable needles.

Magnet therapy

Most claims regarding the healing power of magnets are from manufacturers of products that contain magnets, such as arm and leg wraps, belts, mattress pads and shoe inserts. The manufacturers claim the products can relieve various health problems, including chronic pain, by stimulating your body's natural electrical field.

Although research may someday find magnet therapy to be beneficial, to date there's no scientific evidence that magnets used in this manner provide any health benefits. And some experts believe inappropriate use of magnets could possibly lead to health problems.

A few medical researchers are exploring the use of magnets as a therapy for some forms of chronic pain. Initial reports suggest some possible benefits, but more study is needed. The research also involves different, more powerful magnets, not common refrigerator magnets sold in stores or found in some products.

Tai Chi

Tai Chi (TIE chee) is a form of martial arts developed in China more than 1,000 years ago. No longer used to ward off enemies, it's becoming an increasingly popular method for strengthening muscles, improving flexibility in your joints and reducing stress.

It involves gentle, deliberate circular movements, combined with deep breathing. As you concentrate on the motions of your body, you develop a feeling of tranquility. "Moving meditation" is how Tai Chi is sometimes described. Similar to other forms of Chinese medicine, it's designed to foster the free flow of chi necessary for health.

Most research on Tai Chi has explored its ability to improve your balance and reduce your risk for falls. However, people also report that it helps ease chronic pain by reducing stress and tension.

You can learn Tai Chi from a trained instructor. Classes are also available at some medical and fitness centers.

Therapeutic touch

Therapeutic touch is closely related to the religious concept of laying on of the hands, where healing power is believed to flow from the healer to the patient. However, therapeutic touch isn't based on a religious concept. Instead, it comes from the idea that your body is its own form of energy, surrounded by a field of energy. Illness results when there are disturbances in the surrounding energy field.

Practitioners of therapeutic touch attempt to get rid of these disturbances by moving their hands back and forth across your body. They also believe that by transferring energy from their hands to your body, they can encourage healing and reduce pain, stress and anxiety.

More study is needed to determine if therapeutic touch has any health benefits.

TENS

Transcutaneous electric nerve stimulation (TENS) is prescribed by a doctor. It's intended to relieve pain by preventing pain signals from reaching your brain. TENS is safe and usually painless, but it isn't always effective.

With TENS, small electrodes are placed on your skin, near the area of your pain. The electrodes are attached to a small portable stimulator that you wear. The stimulator delivers tiny electrical impulses through the electrodes to nearby nerve pathways. You turn the TENS unit on and off as needed to control pain.

Exactly how the impulses may relieve pain is uncertain. One theory is that they stimulate production of endorphins, your body's natural painkillers.

TENS generally works best for acute pain associated with a pinched nerve. It's less successful for chronic pain, although some people receive benefit from it. Most often, TENS is used in conjunction with other treatments, including exercise.

A similar and newer procedure under study, called percutaneous electric nerve stimulation (PENS), involves using acupuncturelike needles instead of electrodes to transmit electrical current to your nerves.

Homeopathic and naturopathic medicine

These health care practices don't involve use of traditional medications or surgery. Instead, they attempt to cure and prevent illness through different routes.

Homeopathic medicine

Homeopathic medicine uses highly diluted preparations of natural substances, typically plants and minerals, to treat symptoms of illness. Homeopathy is based on a "law of similars." Practitioners believe that if a large dose of a substance causes you to develop certain symptoms when you're healthy, a small dose of the same substance can treat illnesses that produce the same symptoms.

Working from a list of nearly 2,000 substances, a homeopath selects the most appropriate remedy for your particular set of symptoms. Generally, you take only one "medicine" at a time, until you find one that relieves your symptoms.

Chronic and occasional conditions such as arthritis, asthma, allergies, colds and influenza are the main reasons people use homeopathic medicine. However, some homeopaths believe their remedies can cure all illnesses.

Scientific research isn't able to explain how homeopathic medicines work. And because most homeopathic medicines are so diluted, many modern scientists are skeptical of their effectiveness.

Traditional medical training isn't required to practice homeopathy. However, some homeopaths are physicians, or other types of licensed health professionals, such as chiropractors, nurses or pharmacists. Regulation and licensure of homeopathic practitioners varies from state to state.

Naturopathic medicine

This form of medicine integrates natural therapies, including acupuncture, manipulative therapy, herbal medicines and nutritional therapies, with modern diagnostic sciences and standards of care. Instead of using traditional medications or surgery to treat illness, naturopathic doctors rely on methods aimed at strengthening your body's natural healing ability.

To become certified, naturopathic physicians go through 4 years of medical training. Their training, however, is substantially different from that of traditional medical doctors.

Dietary and herbal remedies

As anyone who's walked through a health food store can attest, the profusion of dietary supplements and herbal remedies is almost overwhelming. Literally thousands of products crowd the shelves, touting all sorts of claims. Two products heavily marketed for pain relief—especially arthritic pain—are:

Dimethyl sulfide. Dimethyl sulfide (DMSO) is an industrial solvent, similar to turpentine. Some people believe that when it's rubbed into your skin it can reduce swelling and pain.

More than 20 years of medical research has produced conflicting results regarding its effectiveness. Doctors generally don't recommend the product for pain relief. Industrial-grade DMSO (sold in hardware stores) may contain poisonous contaminants.

Glucosamine and chondroitin sulfate. These substances claim to help reduce pain by repairing damaged cartilage in your joints. Found naturally in your body, glucosamine is incorporated into substances that give cartilage its strength and rigidity, such as chondroitin, which helps cartilage attract and retain water.

Preliminary evidence suggests glucosamine and chondroitin sulfate supplements may maintain existing cartilage and stimulate growth of new cartilage. But many experts believe large studies are needed to determine whether these supplements offer safe and lasting benefits.

Unlike medications you receive from your doctor, the Food and Drug Administration doesn't regulate the effectiveness of dietary and herbal products. Regulations regarding the safety of these products also are different. With prescription drugs, the manufacturer must prove the benefits of the drug outweigh any safety concerns before the drug is approved for sale. Dietary and herbal supplements, however, are assumed to be safe until they're proven otherwise. Only when a supplement is found unsafe is it removed from the market. In addition, because these products don't follow the same safety procedures, they can contain toxic substances that may not be listed on the label.

The best advice is to talk with your doctor before taking any dietary or herbal product.

Naturopathic physicians claim they can treat the same range of conditions as conventional doctors. However, these claims have not been scientifically proven.

How to approach nontraditional therapies

If you're considering using a complementary or alternative therapy, practice or product—or you already are—the National Center for Complementary and Alternative Medicine recommends these steps:

Research the product or therapy's safety and effectiveness. The benefits you receive from the treatment should outweigh its risks. To find out more about a product or therapy, you can request information from the National Center for Complementary and Alternative Medicine or visit its Web site (see page 169). You also can search for scientific literature on the product or therapy at a public or university library, or via the Internet.

Determine the expertise of the practitioner or salesperson. If you're working with a licensed practitioner, check with your local and state medical boards for information about the person's credentials and whether any complaints have been filed against that person. If you're buying a product from a business or salesperson, check with your local or state business bureau to find out whether any complaints have been filed against the company represented.

Estimate the total cost of the treatment. Because many complementary and alternative approaches aren't covered by health insurance, it's important you know exactly how much the treatment will cost.

Talk with your doctor. Your doctor can help you determine if the treatment may be beneficial and if it's safe. Some complementary and alternative products or therapies may interfere with medications you're taking or negatively affect other health conditions you may have.

Don't substitute a proven treatment for an unproven one. If it's proven that medication or other treatments recommended by your doctor can help your condition, don't replace these treatments with alternative products, practices or therapies that haven't been proven effective.

Chapter 14

Pain Centers and Clinics

S ometimes, major changes in life require personal guidance. If you feel you might benefit from more individualized care, consider visiting a facility that specializes in pain management. There, you can benefit from the knowledge of professionals who deal with chronic pain on a daily basis.

It's a good idea, though, to do a little homework before you make an appointment. Virtually any health care professional can put up a sign and print letterhead that says "Pain Center"or "Pain Clinic." Make sure the professionals you see are reputable and the services they provide are what you really need.

Types of pain programs

Selecting a pain center or pain clinic often means deciding between a specialized or comprehensive approach to pain management. Specialized programs typically focus on a specific method for treating your pain. That method varies according to the facility and the qualifications of the staff. Some specialized programs emphasize use of medication for pain treatment. Others focus on physical therapy or alternative therapies.

If you know the specific cause of your pain, a specialized program may be beneficial. For most people with chronic pain, however, a comprehensive approach to pain management is often the most effective.

A comprehensive approach is the philosophy behind pain management at Mayo Clinic—and the format on which this book is based.

Comprehensive programs encompass the belief that chronic pain affects many aspects of your life and, therefore, requires a broad treatment approach. These programs explore various ways to help you control your pain. In the process, they also help you identify factors in your life that may be contributing to your pain, or making it more difficult to manage. Often, but not always, comprehensive pain programs are associated with medical schools or large medical centers.

At Mayo Clinic, pain specialists integrate behavioral and lifestyle changes with physical and occupational therapy and selective use of medications or injections. Depending on the location or cause of your pain, other therapies, such as biofeedback or TENS, also may be incorporated into your treatment plan.

Research on comprehensive pain programs is positive. It shows that people who take part in a comprehensive program generally get more relief from their pain and have an improved outlook on life than people who receive a single form of therapy or none at all. People in comprehensive programs also are twice as likely to return to work, generally feel less need to visit doctors or other health care providers and typically maintain their progress over long periods.

The pain team

The staff who make up comprehensive pain programs vary. But most programs include some or all of these key professionals:

Physicians
Typically, a physician who has extensive training in the area of chronic pain heads up the team, providing coordination and direction. This person may be a family practitioner or trained in one of several medical specialties, such as neurology, psychiatry, anesthesiology or physiatry (physical medicine and rehabilitation). Just one or a group of doctors may work at the center or clinic.

Psychologists
Psychologists help sort through and address the many behavioral and emotional issues that can accompany chronic pain, such as depression,

anger and fear. They also help pinpoint issues that may be contributing to your pain, such as strained relations with family members or stress at work.

In addition, psychologists teach important skills such as stress reduction and relaxation techniques.

Nurses

Nurses help monitor use of medications or medication withdrawal. They provide information on various treatments and monitor your progress. In many programs, nurses act as "case managers," serving as advocates for you and your family and acting as an intermediary to other professionals on the team. A nurse may be the team member you interact with most often.

Physical and occupational therapists

Therapists are vital to the task of rebuilding your strength, endurance and confidence in your ability to function in the "real world."

Physical therapists do this through their individualized instruction for a complete fitness program. Occupational therapists bolster your independence by focusing on increasing competency in specific, day-to-day tasks. Instruction on proper body mechanics and self-care for sore muscles and stiff joints also are goals of physical and occupational therapy.

Others

Other professionals that may be part of the pain team include:
- A registered dietitian to help you eat more nutritiously and control your weight
- A social worker to help you deal with financial, work, educational or family concerns
- A vocational counselor to help you develop the skills you need to return to work or keep your job
- A recreational therapist to help you safely take part in various recreational activities
- A chaplain to assist with religious and family issues

What to expect

Not all comprehensive pain programs operate exactly the same, but their approach is often quite similar.

Once you've been admitted, you'll receive a thorough evaluation. This may include having the staff review your physical and psychological condition, your use of medication, your work situation and your relationship with your family. The evaluation helps staff devise a treatment plan and personal goals that address your specific problems. These goals might include helping you get off your medication, return to work, become more physically active or learn to relax.

In some programs, the therapy and attention you receive are intensive. You spend most of your day at the center for about 2 to 4 weeks. During this time you work with physical and occupational therapists and spend time in group sessions discussing many of the lifestyle issues outlined in this book. You also meet daily with your case manager to discuss your progress and areas that remain difficult for you.

With other programs, the schedule is more relaxed. You meet for just a few hours each week over several weeks.

How to locate a pain facility

To find a reputable pain program that fits your needs, talk with your doctor. Some programs require a letter of referral from your doctor and a copy of your medical records.

If you have a medical school nearby, check to see if it operates a pain center or clinic. Or, if you're attending a support group, you can ask members of the group if they've been to a pain facility and listen to what they have to say about the program.

You also can receive a list of approved pain centers from the Commission on Accreditation of Rehabilitation Facilities, the organization that certifies pain rehabilitation centers. Other organizations that you can contact for references include the American Pain Society or the American Academy of Pain Medicine. Addresses and phone numbers for these organizations are listed on pages 167 and 168.

What to look for

Pain centers and pain clinics abound. But because facilities and personnel vary in their qualifications and focus, consider these factors when evaluating your options:

Inpatient or outpatient?

When selecting a comprehensive pain program you may need to consider whether you want to take part in the program as an outpatient or as an inpatient (staying at the facility over the course of your treatment). Both approaches have inherent benefits and disadvantages.

The inpatient approach can be beneficial because you're with staff members who can constantly keep a lookout for your negative pain behaviors and help you work on them in a constructive way. The extra support an inpatient clinic offers also can be advantageous if you need to wean yourself from addictive medications.

However, because of this intense, 24-hour-a-day approach, inpatient pain programs generally are more expensive than outpatient programs.

An outpatient pain center provides most or all of the same services as an inpatient program. But you're at the center only during the day—spending nights and weekends at home or at some other accommodation.

The advantage of outpatient programs is that the cost is usually lower. They also give you time away to be with family or at work. However, outpatient programs often run for a longer period than inpatient ones. And if you don't live close to the facility, you may need to pay for overnight accommodations during the length of your stay.

Sometimes, people with an addiction to pain-killing medications start out in an inpatient facility and then transfer to an outpatient program to continue treatment.

What are its goals? Is the program focused simply on relieving your pain, or does it include services to help determine the cause of your pain or personal problems that may be associated with your pain?

What methods does it advocate? Be particularly careful in evaluating programs that advocate long-term use of potentially addictive drugs, such as narcotics, or that routinely include surgery or rely on unproven therapies, such as homeopathy or herbal supplements.

Is the staff friendly and willing to listen? It's important that you feel comfortable with those around you. Members of the staff should be interested in you and your condition and take time to listen to your concerns.

Is the program accredited or certified? It's not required that pain centers or clinics be accredited or certified to operate. However, some states require accreditation to receive insurance reimbursement. Certification also helps ensure the program meets the basic requirements for appropriate medical care.

Does it have a good success rate? Ask what the long-term success rate of the program is. No program can offer a 100 percent success rate. However, generally about half of people who visit comprehensive pain centers are able to return to work.

Does it include follow-up services? If you need additional care once you've completed your treatment, there should be a number you can call or person you can contact. Avoid programs that offer no follow-up care.

How much does it cost? Cost is always a concern. Make sure you know approximately how much the treatment will cost beforehand. And check with your insurance company to see what expenses will be covered. Some insurance companies cover treatment provided by comprehensive pain programs, others don't. And depending on the type of treatment offered, services associated with specialized pain facilities may or may not be covered.

Your role

Pain centers and clinics are similar to the benefits of this book. You can only get from the program what you're willing to put into it. If you're unwilling to learn new skills and you continue to have a negative attitude, the program may help you very little. But if you go into the program with a positive attitude and realistic expectations, you can come away with a better understanding of what you need to do to manage your pain, and confidence in your ability to do it.

Chapter 15

How to Stay in Control

Throughout this book you've read about ways to help lessen your pain and improve your quality of life. Perhaps you've already begun incorporating these changes into your daily routine. But do you worry about what may happen weeks or months from now? How do you maintain the progress you're making? What happens when you're confronted with a "difficult day"?

No doubt, you will have difficult days. And there may be times when you catch yourself reverting to old habits. No one is perfect. However, you can lessen the effects of these occasional setbacks by developing strategies that help keep you on course to an active and rewarding life.

10 ways to maintain your gains

The best advice for staying in control of your pain is to regularly use the pain management strategies outlined in this book, such as exercise, moderation and relaxation. The more you use them, the more beneficial they'll become.

To maintain your progress and avoid relapses:

1. Follow through on your goals
Select your areas of greatest concern, then set some specific, measurable

and realistic goals to help you deal with those issues. You might be worried, for example, that you'll slip back into your old pain behaviors, such as moaning, complaining or limping. Or, maybe, you're concerned about keeping up your exercise program.

Create a checklist, and put an X by each goal you reach. To help strengthen your motivation, ask a family member or a friend to periodically review your checklist.

2. Monitor your progress
Seeing the accomplishments you've made can motivate you to continue your goals. Use charts or some way to display your progress.

3. Write yourself a contract
Some people find that making a personal commitment to improving their lives and managing their pain helps them follow through on their plans. More than just a goal, this contract becomes a pledge associated with other binding agreements you've made throughout your life.

4. Plan your day
When you specifically schedule time for something—such as exercise or going to a movie—you're more likely to do it. Also use "to-do" lists or notes on a calendar to remind you of your priorities.

5. Keep your surroundings healthful
Look around your house and get rid of things that might lure you back into unhealthful habits. For example, is your bed still sitting in the living room to avoid having to walk upstairs to your bedroom? Are the drapes pulled to keep your rooms dark? Make your house feel like a home, not a hospital or a mortuary. When you walk around your house, you want to see evidence of a person who lives a happy and active life.

6. Seek and accept support
Accepting help from others isn't a sign of weakness, nor does it mean that you're failing. You need support from others to keep you on track and to help you when you have difficult days. In addition to support from family and friends, consider joining a chronic pain support group. These groups are discussed further on page 155.

7. Work with your doctor

Your doctor can be one of your biggest advocates. Keep your doctor updated on your progress and any obstacles you may encounter. He or she can often help you overcome those obstacles.

8. Stay positive

List as many positive statements about yourself as you can and say them to yourself when you're feeling discouraged or in danger of slipping back into some of your old patterns of unhealthful behavior.

If you do have a relapse, accept that it happens, and move on again, positively.

9. Prepare for challenging situations

Make a list of situations that could disrupt the positive lifestyle changes you've made. Whatever they are, prepare a response plan that you can activate when needed.

Perhaps you've been walking for 30 minutes each day, but you know the weather will soon be changing and you don't like being outside in the snow or cold. How do you still fit in your 30-minute walk each day? One option might be to walk indoors at a nearby mall. Or, perhaps, a local school allows indoor walking during certain hours. You might also consider purchasing a treadmill.

Another example might be a change at work. You know that in one month your job is going to change and that you'll be taking on some new responsibilities. That worries you. One way you might make the transition easier is by developing a list ahead of time. Write down all of the new things you'll need to learn. Prioritize which is the most important and then decide what steps you need to take to learn each task. Knowing ahead of time exactly what you need to do and how you're going to do it will make the transition less stressful.

10. Reward yourself

Rewards are a great way to reinforce positive change. When you reach a goal, or successfully execute one of your pain strategies, treat yourself to something enjoyable. That might include a relaxing cup of tea following your daily walk or attending a sporting event for completing your 6-month stress reduction goal.

Getting through a difficult day

Everyone has a bad day now and then. Holidays can be difficult. Then there's bill time, or an unpredicted 10-inch snowfall overnight. A visit from relatives may also qualify.

Whatever the reason for your bad day, you can get through it. One of the best ways to minimize the disruptiveness of a tough day and quickly get back to your usual activities is to plan for it. The time to plan for a difficult day is when you're having a good day. On a bad day, it's often difficult to think of ways to cope with the problem. In fact, it can be challenging to concentrate on much of anything except the reason behind the day's souring effect.

Here's how to plan ahead for a difficult day:

Identify sources of your difficult days. Knowing the most common reasons for your difficult days will help you better prepare for them. Think about some recent bad days. Was there a reason for your increased pain? Could it be from too much stress, overdoing it on the weekends, traveling or lack of exercise?

Identify your warning signs. Do you get a warning sign a bad day is headed your way, such as a headache, excessive fatigue or onset of the "blues"?

Develop a game plan. When you know a difficult day is coming, or you get a warning sign, you can lessen its effects by structuring that day with activities and diversions. Your game plan may include some of the following strategies:

Maintain a normal schedule. A difficult day is not a time to overdo it—or to do nothing. Lying around won't help your pain improve or the day go by any faster.

Get out of the house. When you're hurting, it's natural to want to be alone and tend your wounds. But this only gives you more opportunity to think about your pain. Go shopping or visit a friend who can keep you occupied. But steer your conversations away from your pain.

Seek other diversions. Read something enjoyable. Watch a funny movie or call a friend who has a good sense of humor.

Try to relax. On a difficult day, spend more time practicing your relaxation techniques, such as listening to soothing tapes or practicing your breathing exercises.

Keep away from medication. If you've weaned yourself from medication, don't let a bad day tempt you into taking it again. Remind yourself that it's only a temporary solution and that you're better off without it. If you're taking medication, don't change the dose in an attempt to reduce the pain. You only increase your risk for side effects, and the increased dose may not help your pain.

Say, "This will pass." Because it will.

Joining a support group

More than 15 million Americans with chronic pain regularly attend support group meetings. These groups can provide a depth of help and advice and a sense of control that you might not find anywhere else. That's because they put you face-to-face with people who share many of the same symptoms and feelings as you do.

Not all support groups are the same. Some support groups are mostly educational and feature discussions led by informed guest speakers. Others are more social and unstructured, with meetings providing a time to vent, brag, encourage and visit. No matter how the groups are set up, they all share the same basic goal: to help each member cope with his or her pain.

What support groups offer

Benefits of support groups include:

A sense of belonging, of fitting in. There's a special bond among people whose lives have been disrupted by the same problem. You share a sense of camaraderie. Once you experience how others accept you just as you are, you begin to feel more accepting toward yourself.

People who understand what you're going through. Family, friends and doctors can sympathize with your problems, but they often can't empathize because they haven't experienced what you have. Your pain experience is unique, but it shares many common threads. Support group members have a good idea of what you're feeling and experiencing. Because of this, you feel freer to speak your mind and voice your frustrations, disappointments and anger.

Exchange of advice. You may be skeptical of some of the advice well-meaning friends give you, because they don't have chronic pain. But when veteran group members talk, you know they speak with the voice of first-hand experience. They can tell you about coping techniques that have worked wonders for them—and techniques that haven't helped at all.

Opportunity to make new friends. These friends can bring joy into your life as well as practical support: a listening ear when you need to talk, a chauffeur when you could use a relaxing drive and a companion to exercise with.

When support groups aren't the answer

Support groups aren't for everyone. To gain the most benefit from a group setting you have to be willing to share your thoughts and feelings. You also must be willing to learn about and help others. People who are severely depressed and don't want to talk or who have poor social skills are generally less likely to benefit from support groups.

In addition, not all support groups are beneficial. You want to be in a group where the mood is upbeat and the message positive. Some groups that aren't carefully monitored can become a place to vent and share only negative feelings that breed on themselves. This can leave you depressed and add to your pain instead of improve it.

How to find a support group

Your community may already have one or more support groups for people with chronic pain. There may even be groups for specific types of chronic pain, such as arthritis, fibromyalgia or irritable bowel syndrome.

To find out if there's a support group in your community, check with your doctor or nurse. You might also check with your county health department, a community health organization or your local library. You can also contact organizations such as the American Chronic Pain Association or the National Chronic Pain Outreach Association. These agencies offer free information on area support groups. They also can provide information and advice on how to start a support group if there isn't one in your community. The addresses and phone numbers for the agencies are listed on pages 167 and 169.

It's up to you

We wrote this book to help you better understand how pain works and to identify effective techniques that can help control pain. The rest is up to you.

Our hope is that you can incorporate some or all of the suggestions in this book into your daily life. We believe the more active and productive you can become, the happier you'll be and the better you'll feel. With the right skills and attitude, there's no limit to how much you can accomplish.

Your Personal Planner

Planning your day can help you find a more healthful balance to your daily routine. Use the daily planners that follow to schedule your day from the time you wake up until you go to bed. You can plan a day at a time or make your plans for an entire week.

Each day, include a mixture of work, rest, exercise, relaxation and social activities. If you have trouble fitting everything in, ask yourself these three questions:

What do I *have* **to do today?** That might include going to work, making it to a scheduled appointment or getting some exercise.

What would be *best done* **today?** These are things you don't have to do, but will need your attention at some point. This might include doing a load of laundry, catching up on your bookwork or completing a project at work. Instead of having these activities pile up, it's best to try to spread them out over the week.

What do I *want* **to do today?** It's important to spend a certain amount of time each day doing things you enjoy and that help you relax. This could be working in your flower bed, playing a round of golf, visiting with a friend or reading a good book.

Include at least one response to each of these questions as you plan your day. If you're unsure of your plans on certain days, mark as best you can what you think you may be doing. To help you stay on track, refer to your planner throughout the day. Periodically write down what you did and compare it with your plan.

If you find that scheduling your day helps you to achieve your goals, then continue to do so. You can purchase a daily planner in most office supply and many discount stores. Or, you can make your own. However, once you get into a routine, you may find that you don't need to be as detailed in your planning. Marking down a few key times or events may be all you need.

On the following page is a sample day to give you an idea of the information you might include in your daily schedule.

Day: _____*Thursday*_____

Date: _____*January 6*_____

	I plan to	**I did**
6:00 a.m.	*Wake up, exercise, have breakfast*	*Exercised, had breakfast*
7:00 a.m.	*Clean up and leave for work*	*Got ready and went to work*
8:00 a.m.	*Finish letters from yesterday*	*Letters*
9:00 a.m.	*Complete letters*	*Letters, worked on meeting agenda*
10:00 a.m.	*Start work on new files*	*Letters*
11:00 a.m.	*New files*	*Started new files*
12:00 p.m.	*Meet Susan for lunch*	*Lunch with Susan*
1:00 p.m.	*Continue work on files*	*New files*
2:00 p.m.	*Department meeting*	*Meeting*
3:00 p.m.	*Complete files*	*Meeting follow-up*
4:00 p.m.	*Make phone calls, other details*	*Phone calls, memos, etc.*
5:00 p.m.	*Go home, rest, ride bike*	*Went home, rested, rode bike*
6:00 p.m.	*Prepare and eat dinner*	*Dinner*
7:00 p.m.	*Do laundry and iron*	*Laundry, rested*
8:00 p.m.	*Work on class reunion schedule*	*Ironed, visited with Connie*
9:00 p.m.	*Relaxation exercises, rest*	*Relaxation exercises, helped Al*
10:00 p.m.	*Read book, go to bed*	*Read book and went to bed*
11:00 p.m.	*Sleep*	*Slept*

Day: _____

Date: _____

	I plan to	I did
6:00 a.m.		
7:00 a.m.		
8:00 a.m.		
9:00 a.m.		
10:00 a.m.		
11:00 a.m.		
12:00 p.m.		
1:00 p.m.		
2:00 p.m.		
3:00 p.m.		
4:00 p.m.		
5:00 p.m.		
6:00 p.m.		
7:00 p.m.		
8:00 p.m.		
9:00 p.m.		
10:00 p.m.		
11:00 p.m.		

PERSONAL PLANNER

Day: _____

Date: _____

	I plan to	I did
6:00 a.m.		
7:00 a.m.		
8:00 a.m.		
9:00 a.m.		
10:00 a.m.		
11:00 a.m.		
12:00 p.m.		
1:00 p.m.		
2:00 p.m.		
3:00 p.m.		
4:00 p.m.		
5:00 p.m.		
6:00 p.m.		
7:00 p.m.		
8:00 p.m.		
9:00 p.m.		
10:00 p.m.		
11:00 p.m.		

PERSONAL PLANNER

Day: _____

Date: _____

	I plan to	I did
6:00 a.m.		
7:00 a.m.		
8:00 a.m.		
9:00 a.m.		
10:00 a.m.		
11:00 a.m.		
12:00 p.m.		
1:00 p.m.		
2:00 p.m.		
3:00 p.m.		
4:00 p.m.		
5:00 p.m.		
6:00 p.m.		
7:00 p.m.		
8:00 p.m.		
9:00 p.m.		
10:00 p.m.		
11:00 p.m.		

PERSONAL **PLANNER**

Day: _____

Date: _____

	I plan to	I did
6:00 a.m.		
7:00 a.m.		
8:00 a.m.		
9:00 a.m.		
10:00 a.m.		
11:00 a.m.		
12:00 p.m.		
1:00 p.m.		
2:00 p.m.		
3:00 p.m.		
4:00 p.m.		
5:00 p.m.		
6:00 p.m.		
7:00 p.m.		
8:00 p.m.		
9:00 p.m.		
10:00 p.m.		
11:00 p.m.		

P
E
R
S
O
N
A
L

**P
L
A
N
N
E
R**

Day: _____

Date: _____

	I plan to	I did
6:00 a.m.		
7:00 a.m.		
8:00 a.m.		
9:00 a.m.		
10:00 a.m.		
11:00 a.m.		
12:00 p.m.		
1:00 p.m.		
2:00 p.m.		
3:00 p.m.		
4:00 p.m.		
5:00 p.m.		
6:00 p.m.		
7:00 p.m.		
8:00 p.m.		
9:00 p.m.		
10:00 p.m.		
11:00 p.m.		

PERSONAL **PLANNER**

Day: _____

Date: _____

	I plan to	I did
6:00 a.m.		
7:00 a.m.		
8:00 a.m.		
9:00 a.m.		
10:00 a.m.		
11:00 a.m.		
12:00 p.m.		
1:00 p.m.		
2:00 p.m.		
3:00 p.m.		
4:00 p.m.		
5:00 p.m.		
6:00 p.m.		
7:00 p.m.		
8:00 p.m.		
9:00 p.m.		
10:00 p.m.		
11:00 p.m.		

Day: _____

Date: _____

	I plan to	I did
6:00 a.m.		
7:00 a.m.		
8:00 a.m.		
9:00 a.m.		
10:00 a.m.		
11:00 a.m.		
12:00 p.m.		
1:00 p.m.		
2:00 p.m.		
3:00 p.m.		
4:00 p.m.		
5:00 p.m.		
6:00 p.m.		
7:00 p.m.		
8:00 p.m.		
9:00 p.m.		
10:00 p.m.		
11:00 p.m.		

PERSONAL PLANNER

Day: _____

Date: _____

	I plan to	I did
6:00 a.m.		
7:00 a.m.		
8:00 a.m.		
9:00 a.m.		
10:00 a.m.		
11:00 a.m.		
12:00 p.m.		
1:00 p.m.		
2:00 p.m.		
3:00 p.m.		
4:00 p.m.		
5:00 p.m.		
6:00 p.m.		
7:00 p.m.		
8:00 p.m.		
9:00 p.m.		
10:00 p.m.		
11:00 p.m.		

Additional Resources

Contact these organizations for more information about chronic pain or associated conditions. Some groups offer free printed material or videos. Others have material or videos you can purchase.

American Academy of Head, Neck and Facial Pain
520 West Pipeline Road
Hurst, Texas 76053
817-282-1501
Fax: 817-282-8012
Web site: *www.aahnfp.org*

American Academy of Orofacial Pain
19 Mantua Road
Mount Royal, NJ 08061
856-423-3629
Fax: 856-423-3420
Web site: *www.aaop.org*

American Academy of Pain Medicine
4700 West Lake Avenue
Glenview, IL 60025
847-375-4731
Fax: 847-375-4777
Web site: *www.painmed.org*

American Art Therapy Association
1202 Allanson Road
Mundelein, IL 60060-3808
847-949-6064
Fax: 847-566-4580
Web site: *www.arttherapy.org*

American Chronic Pain Association
P.O. Box 850
Rocklin, CA 95677-0850
916-632-0922
Fax: 916-632-3208
Web site: *www.theacpa.org*

American Council for Headache Education
19 Mantua Road
Mount Royal, NJ 08061
800-255-2243
609-423-0258
Fax: 609-423-0082
Web site: *www.achenet.org*

American Dance Therapy Association
10632 Little Patuxent Parkway
2000 Century Plaza, Suite 108
Columbia, MD 21044
410-997-4040
Fax: 410-997-4048

American Fibromyalgia Syndrome Association, Inc.
6380 East Tanque Verde, Suite D
Tucson, AZ 85715
520-733-1570
Fax: 520-290-5550
Web site: *www.afsafund.org*

American Music Therapy Association
8455 Colesville Road, Suite 1000
Silver Spring, MD 20910
301-589-3300
Fax: 301-589-5175
Web site: *www.musictherapy.org*

American Pain Foundation
111 South Calvert Street
Suite 2700
Baltimore, MD 21202
Web site: *www.painfoundation.org*

American Pain Society
4700 West Lake Avenue
Glenview, IL 60025-1485
847-375-4715
Fax: 847-375-4777
Web site: *www.ampainsoc.org*

Arthritis Foundation
1330 West Peachtree Street
Atlanta, GA 30309
800-283-7800
404-872-7100
Fax: 404-872-0457
Web site: *www.arthritis.org*

Commission on Accreditation of Rehabilitation Facilities
4891 East Grant Rd.
Tucson, AZ 85712
800-444-8991
520-325-1044
Fax: 520-318-1129
Web site: *www.carf.org*

Endometriosis Association
8585 North 76th Place
Milwaukee, WI 53223
414-355-2200
Fax: 414-355-6065
Web site: *www.endometriosisassn.org*

Fibromyalgia Network
P.O. Box 31750
Tucson, AZ 85751-1750
800-853-2929
Fax: 520-290-5550
Web site: *www.fmnetnews.com*

**International Association for
the Study of Pain**
909 Northeast 43rd Street
Suite 306
Seattle, WA 98105-6020
206-547-6409
Fax: 206-547-1703
Web site: *www.halcyon.com/iasp*

**International Foundation
for Functional
Gastrointestinal Disorders**
P.O. Box 17864
Milwaukee, WI 53217
888-964-2001
Web site: *www.iffgd.org*

Interstitial Cystitis Association
51 Monroe Street, Suite 1402
Rockville, MD 20850
301-610-5300
Fax: 301-610-5308
Web site: *www.ichelp.org*

**JAMA Migraine Information Center,
The Journal of the American
Medical Association**
Web site: *www.ama-assn.org/
special/migraine/newsline*

Mayo Clinic Health Oasis
Web site: *www.mayohealth.org*

**National Center for Complementary
and Alternative Medicine**
888-644-6226
Web site: *nccam.nih.gov*

**National Chronic Pain
Outreach Association**
7979 Old Georgetown Road
Suite 100
Bethesda, MD 20814-2429
301-652-4948
301-698-5452

National Headache Foundation
428 West St. James Place, 2nd Floor
Chicago, IL 60614
800-843-2256
773-388-6399
Fax: 773-525-7357
Web site: *www.headaches.org*

Neuropathy Association
60 East 42nd Street
Suite 942
New York, NY 10165-0999
212-692-0662
Fax: 212-692-0668
Web site: *www.neuropathy.org*

**Reflex Sympathetic Dystrophy
Syndrome Association**
116 Haddon Avenue, Suite D
Haddonfield, NJ 08033
609-795-8845
Web site: *www.rsds.org*

TMJ Association, Ltd
P.O. Box 26770
Milwaukee, WI 53226-0770
414-259-3223
Fax: 414-259-8112
Web site: *www.tmj.org*

Trigeminal Neuralgia Association
P.O. Box 340
Barnegat Light, NJ 08006
609-361-1014
Fax: 609-361-0982
Web site: *neurosurgery.mgh.
harvard.edu/tna*

Index

A

Abdominal exercises, 60–61
Acetaminophen, 121
Achilles tendon stretch, 56
Activity level
    decrease, 27
    exercise program, 53–66
    fluctuations, 25–26
    keeping a journal, 44–46
    moderation, 66, 70–71
    overdoing it, 27, 67
    rest periods, 71
    setting goals, 47–48
Acupressure, 139
Acupuncture, 139–140
Acute pain, 6, 24
Addiction, 40, 124
Additional resources, 167-170
Aerobic exercise, 58–59
Aggressive behavior, 84
Alcohol
    and acetaminophen, 121
    and medications, 40, 111, 121
    and migraine, 17
    moderate drinking, 111
    and sleep problems, 36, 103
Alternative medicine, 133–144
Analgesics
    acetaminophen, 121
    aspirin, 120
    cox-2 inhibitors, 121
    NSAIDs, 120
    ointments, 122
    rebound pain, 123
Anger, 30, 78–79
Ankle flexibility exercises, 56
Anti-seizure medications, 126
Antidepressants
    for pain relief, 125, 126–127
    and sexual performance, 116
    side effects, 125
    as sleep aids, 104, 128

Anxiety, 36–37
Arm exercises, 63
Aromatherapy, 137
Art therapy, 136
Arthritis, 9–11
Aspirin, 120
Aspirin ointments, 122
Assertiveness, 84–85
Autonomic nerves, 3, 5

B

Back exercises, 61
Back pain, 1, 10, 11–13
    and chiropractic, 137
Back stretch, 58
Balancing your day, 67–71
Biofeedback, 134
Body mass index (BMI), 105–106
Body mechanics and movement,
    72–75
Brain and pain signals, 4–5
Breathing during exertion, 74

C

Caffeine and sleep problems, 103
Cancer pain, 24
Capsaicin ointments, 122
Carpal tunnel syndrome, 22
Catastrophizing problems, 82
Central nervous system, 3
Certified exercise therapist, 58
Chemical dependency, 39–40
Chest exercises, 63
Chiropractic manipulation, 137
Chondroitin sulfate, 143
Choosing a doctor, 42
Chronic pain
    behavioral cycle, 25–27, 34
    causes of, 7, 9–24
    costs of, 35–40, 78
    defined, 1
    difficult days, 154–155

Chronic pain — cont'd
    emotional cycle, 28–31, 34
    family responses, 31–33
    incidence, 7
    information sources, 43
    medication crutch, 132
    pain clinics, 145–150
    psychological factors, 24
    taking control, 41–52
Cluster headache, 18
Cold therapy, 131
Communication skills, 97–98
Complementary medicine, 133–144
Complex regional pain syndrome
    (CRPS), 13–14, 130
Coping skills, 8, 41–52, 154–155
Cox-2 inhibitors, 121
Cyclooxygenase, 120, 121

D
Daily planner, 69, 157-166
Dance therapy, 136
Deconditioning, 27, 35–36
Deep breathing, 92–93
Depression
    chemical imbalance, 126
    and chronic pain, 31, 37, 78
    symptoms of, 37–38
Diabetic neuropathy, 122
Dietary remedies, 143
Difficult days, 154–155
Dimethyl sulfide (DMSO), 143
Doctor, choosing, 42
Drugs. see Medications
Drugs, illicit, 39–40

E
Elbow flexibility exercises, 55
Emotional upheaval
    and chemical dependency, 40
    with chronic pain, 36–37, 77–86
    expressing feelings, 97–98,
        155–156
Emotionalizing, 82
Endometriosis, 14
Endorphins, 4

Enkephalins, 4
Exercise
    aerobic, 58–59
    flexibility, 54–56
    goal setting, 47–48, 65
    motivation, 65–66
    Perceived Exertion Scale, 59
    posture, 63–65
    and sound sleep, 103
    strengthening, 60–63
    and stress reduction, 90
    stretching, 56–58
    variety, 66

F
Facial pain. see Orofacial pain
Family relationships
    behavioral cycle, 32–33
    emotional cycle, 32–33
    goal setting, 47–48, 50
    health benefits, 95–96
    helpful suggestions, 99–100
    strains, 39
    time demands, 69
Feldenkrais, 138
Fibromyalgia, 15
Filtering experiences, 82
Financial strain, 38–39
Finger flexibility exercises, 55
Fitness program, 53–66
Flares, 45, 130, 132
Flexibility exercises, 54–56
Foot flexibility exercises, 56
Friends and family, 32–33, 39,
        95–100

G
Getting organized, 70, 89
Glucosamine, 143
Goal setting, 47–52, 65
    maintaining goals, 151–153
Groaning and grimacing, 28
Guided imagery, 93

H
Hamstring stretch, 57

Headache, 16–18. *See also* Migraine
Health care professionals
    certified exercise therapist, 58
    nurse, 147
    occupational therapist, 58, 147
    osteopath, 138
    pain specialist, 42, 146
    physical therapist, 58, 147
    physician, 42, 146
    psychologist, 146–147
Health clubs, 58
Healthy eating, 108–111
Heat therapy, 131
Heel cord stretch, 56
Herbal remedies, 143
Herniated disk, 13
Hip flexibility exercises, 56
Hip flexor stretch, 57
Homeopathic medicine, 142
Housework tips, 70, 72
Humor therapy, 134–135
Hypnosis, 135

I
Ibuprofen, 120
Ice massage, 131
Immune system
    and hope, 117
    and inactivity, 36
    and rheumatoid arthritis, 11
    and self-esteem, 85
    and social connections, 95
    and stress, 88
Inactivity
    and immune system, 36
    and osteoporosis risk, 36
    and physical deconditioning, 35–36
    and sleep problems, 36
Injections for pain, 130, 132
Injuries, 4, 5
Internet information sources, 43
Interstitial cystitis, 18–19
Intimacy, 115
Irritable bowel syndrome, 19
Isolation, 27, 67
    goal setting, 47–48, 50

J
Jaw flexibility exercises, 55
Jaw pain. *See* Orofacial pain
Journal, 43–46

K
Keeping a journal, 43–46
Ketoprofen, 120
Kneeling, 73

L
Laughter and pain reduction, 134–135
Leg exercises, 62
Lidocaine, 127
Lifting properly, 74
Limbic center and pain perception, 5
Limping, 28
Lithium, 128
Losing weight, 107–108
Low back pain. *See* Back pain
Low back stretch, 58

M
Magnet therapy, 140
Massage therapy, 137–138
Mayo Clinic Health Oasis, 129
Medications, 119-132
    acetaminophen, 121
    Actron (ketoprofen), 120
    Advil (ibuprofen), 120
    Aleve (naproxen sodium), 120
    alprazolam, 129
    Ambien (zolpidem), 129
    Amerge (naratriptan), 127
    amitriptyline, 125
    amoxapine, 125
    Anacin-3 (acetaminophen), 121
    Anafranil (clomipramine), 125
    analgesics, 119–122
    Anaprox DS (naproxen), 120
    Ansaid (flurbiprofen), 120
    anti-seizure medications, 126
    ArthriCare, 122
    Asendin (amoxapine), 125
    Aspercreme (trolamine
        salicylate), 122

Medications — cont'd
aspirin, 120
Aspirin-Free Anacin
(acetaminophen), 121
Aspirin-Free Excedrin
(acetaminophen), 121
aspirin ointments, 122
Ativan (lorazepam), 129
Aventyl (nortriptyline), 125
baclofen, 129
Ben-Gay, 122
bupropion, 113, 128
butabarbital sodium, 129
Butisol Sodium (butabarbital
sodium), 129
butorphanol, 123
capsaicin ointments, 122
Capzasin-P (capsaicin), 122
carbamazepine, 126, 128
Carbatrol (carbamazepine), 126
carisoprodol, 129
Celebrex (celecoxib), 121
celecoxib, 121
Celexa (citalopram), 128
chlordiazepoxide, 129
chlorzoxazone, 129
citalopram, 128
Clinoril (sulindac), 120
clomipramine, 125
clonazepam, 129
clorazepate, 129
codeine, 123
as a crutch, 132
cyclobenzaprine, 129
cyproheptadine, 127
Dalmane (flurazepam), 129
Darvocet (propoxyphene), 123
Darvon (propoxyphene), 123
Daypro (oxaprozin), 120
Demerol (meperidine), 123
Depakote (valproic acid), 127, 128
desipramine, 125
Desyrel (trazodone), 128
D.H.E. 45 (dihydroergotamine), 127
diazepam, 129
diclofenac sodium, 120

Medications — cont'd
dihydroergotamine, 127
Dilantin (phenytoin), 126
Dilaudid (hydromorphone), 123
Dolophine (methadone), 123
Dolorac (capsaicin), 122
doxepin, 125
Duragesic (fentanyl), 123
Duramorph (morphine), 123
Effexor (venlafaxine), 128
Elavil (amitriptyline), 125
Endep (amitriptyline), 125
Epitol (carbamazepine), 128
Ercaf (ergotamine), 127
Ergomar (ergotamine), 127
ergotamine, 127
Eskalith (lithium), 128
estazolam, 129
etodolac, 120
Excedrin (aspirin), 120
Feldene (piroxicam), 120
fenoprofen, 120
fentanyl, 123
Fioricet, 127
Fiorinal, 127
Flexeril (cyclobenzaprine), 129
fluoxetine, 128
flurazepam, 129
flurbiprofen, 120
fluvoxamine, 128
gabapentin, 126, 128
Halcion (triazolam), 129
hydrocodone, 123
hydromorphone, 123
ibuprofen, 120
Icy Hot, 122
imipramine, 125
Imitrex (sumatriptan), 127
Indocin (indomethacin), 120
indomethacin, 120
injections, 130, 132
ketoprofen, 120
ketorolac tromethamine, 120
Klonopin (clonazepam), 129
Lamictal (lamotrigine), 126
lamotrigine, 126

Medications — cont'd
Levo-Dromoran (levorphanol), 123
levorphanol, 123
Librium (chlordiazepoxide), 129
Lioresal (baclofen), 129
lithium, 128
Lithobid (lithium), 128
Lodine XL (etodolac), 120
long-term use, 119
lorazepam, 129
Lorcet (hydrocodone), 123
Lortab (hydrocodone), 123
Ludiomil (maprotiline), 128
Luvox (fluvoxamine), 128
maprotiline, 128
Maxalt (rizatriptan), 127
meperidine, 123
methadone, 123
methocarbamol, 129
methyl ointments, 122
methysergide, 127
Midrin, 127
mirtazapine, 128
monoamine oxidase inhibitors, 128
morphine, 123
Motrin IB (ibuprofen), 120
MS Contin (morphine), 123
muscle relaxants, 129
Myoflex (trolamine salicylate), 122
nabumetone, 120
Nalfon (fenoprofen), 120
Naprelan (naproxen), 120
Naprosyn (naproxen), 120
naproxen, 120
naproxen sodium, 120
naratriptan, 127
Nardil (phenelzine), 128
nefazodone, 128
Nembutal Sodium (pentobarbital
    sodium), 129
nerve blocks, 130
Neurontin (gabapentin), 126, 128
Norflex (orphenadrine), 129
Norpramin (desipramine), 125
nortriptyline, 125
NSAIDs, 120

Medications — cont'd
Numorphan (oxymorphone), 123
Nuprin (ibuprofen), 120
orphenadrine, 129
Orudis KT (ketoprofen), 120
oxaprozin, 120
oxazepam, 129
oxycodone, 123
oxymorphone, 123
pain pumps, 124
Pamelor (nortriptyline), 125
Panadol (acetaminophen), 121
Parafon Forte (chlorzoxazone), 129
Parnate (tranylcypromine), 128
paroxetine, 128
Paxil (paroxetine), 128
pentobarbital sodium, 129
Percocet (oxycodone), 123
Periactin (cyproheptadine), 127
phenelzine, 128
phenytoin, 126
piroxicam, 120
propoxyphene, 123
ProSom (estazolam), 129
protriptyline, 125
Prozac (fluoxetine), 128
pseudoephedrine, 103
Relafen (nabumetone), 120
Remeron (mirtazapine), 128
rizatriptan, 127
Robaxin (methocarbamol), 129
rofecoxib, 121
Roxanol (morphine), 123
Roxicet (oxycodone), 123
Sansert (methysergide), 127
sedatives, 129
Serax (oxazepam), 129
sertraline, 127
Serzone (nefazodone), 128
and sexual performance, 116
side effects, 120–126, 128, 129, 132
Sinequan (doxepin), 125
and sleep problems, 36, 101, 103
Soma (carisoprodol), 129
Sportscreme (trolamine
    salicylate), 122

Medications — cont'd
  SSRIs, 126, 128
  Stadol (butorphanol), 123
  Sublimaze (fentanyl), 123
  sulindac, 120
  sumatriptan, 127
  Surmontil (trimipramine), 125
  Tegretol (carbamazepine), 126, 128
  Tofranil (imipramine), 125
  Toradol (ketorolac
      tromethamine), 120
  tramadol, 124–125
  Tranxene (clorazepate), 129
  tranylcypromine, 128
  trazodone, 128
  triazolam, 129
  tricyclic antidepressants, 125–126
  trigger-point injections, 130, 132
  trimipramine, 125
  trolamine salicylate, 122
  Tylenol (acetaminophen), 121
  Tylenol with codeine, 123
  Tylox (oxycodone), 123
  Ultram (tramadol), 124–125
  Valium (diazepam), 129
  valproate, 128
  valproic acid, 127
  vasoconstrictors, 127
  venlafaxine, 128
  Vicodin (hydrocodone), 123
  Vioxx (rofecoxib), 121
  Vivactil (protriptyline), 125
  Voltaren XR (diclofenac sodium),
      120
  Wellbutrin (bupropion), 113, 128
  Wigraine (ergotamine), 127
  Xanax (alprazolam), 129
  zolmitriptan, 127
  Zoloft (sertraline), 128
  zolpidem, 129
  Zomig (zolmitriptan), 127
  Zostrix (capsaicin), 122
  Zyban, 113
Meditation, 135–136
Methyl ointments, 122
Migraine, 16–18
  medications, 127

Mind-body connection, 134–136
Moderation, 70–71, 82–83
Modification of tasks, 71–72
Monoamine oxidase inhibitors, 128
Mood changes
  keeping a journal, 45–46
  with pain level, 36–37
Mood-stabilizing medications, 128
Motor nerves, 3
Mouth pain. see Orofacial pain
Movement and body mechanics, 72–75
"Movement" therapies, 138
Muscle relaxants, 129
Muscle spasm
  and back pain, 12
  and neck pain, 21
  and pelvic floor pain, 22–23
Music therapy, 136

N

Naproxen sodium, 120
Naps and sleep problems, 104
Narcotics, 123–125, 132
National Center for Complementary
      and Alternative Medicine,
      133, 144
Natural painkillers, 4
Naturopathic medicine, 142, 144
Neck flexibility exercises, 54–55
Neck pain
  anatomy of, 21
Negative thinking, 81–82
Nerve blocks, 130
Neuroma, 7
Neuropathic pain
  defined, 7
Nicotine and sleep problems, 103
Nicotine replacement, 113
Nociceptors, 2, 3
Nonsteroidal anti-inflammatory
      drugs (NSAIDs), 120
NREM sleep, 102
Nutrition, 108–111

O

Obesity, 105–106
Occupational therapist, 58

Ointments for pain relief, 122
Organization skills, 70, 89
Orofacial pain, 19–21
Osteoarthritis, 10
Osteopathy, 138
Overuse injuries, 22

P

Pain
  acute vs. chronic, 6–7, 24
  anatomy of, 2–5
  cold and heat therapy, 131
  medications, 119–132
  rating level of, 44
  rebound pain, 123
  response to, 5–6
Pain behaviors, 28
  goal setting, 47–49
Pain clinics, 145–150
  choosing, 148–150
  inpatient vs. outpatient, 149
  locating, 148
Pain-enhancers, 4
Pain pumps, 124
Pain-stress cycle, 87
Passive behavior, 83–85
Pelvic floor pain, 22–23
Perceived Exertion Scale, 59
Percutaneous electric nerve
    stimulation (PENS), 141
Perfectionists
  and adjusting expectations, 82–83
  and chronic pain, 31
Peripheral nerve block, 130
Peripheral nerves
  anatomy of, 2–3
Personal planner, 69, 157-166
Personalizing events, 82
Physical therapist, 58
Polarizing situations, 82
Positive thinking, 80–81, 90
Postherpetic neuralgia, 23–24, 122
Posture, 28, 63–65
Problem-solving skills, 90–91
Progressive muscle relaxation, 93
Protective posture, 28
Pushing and pulling properly, 75

Q

Quadriceps stretch, 57
Quitting smoking, 112–114

R

Range-of-motion exercises, 54–56
Rating pain level, 44
Reaching properly, 73
Rebound headache, 18
Rebound pain, 123
Recreation, 68
  goal setting, 47–48, 50
Relaxation
  deep breathing, 92–93
  goal setting, 47–49
  guided imagery, 93
  progressive muscle relaxation, 93
  word repetition, 93
REM sleep, 102
Resources, 167-170
Rheumatoid arthritis, 11
Riboflavin, 127
Rolfing, 139

S

Sciatica, 12
Sedatives, 129
  and sexual performance, 116
Selective serotonin reuptake
    inhibitors (SSRIs), 126, 128
Self-esteem, 31, 85–86
Self-talk, 80–82
Sensory nerves, 3
Serotonin, 126
  and migraine, 17
Sexuality
  alternatives to intercourse, 116
  difficulties with chronic pain, 37,
      39, 114, 115
  experimentation, 116
  non-sexual intimacy, 115
Shingles, 23–24
Shoulder flexibility exercises, 55
Sleep
  and chronic pain, 36, 101–102
  improving, 103–104
  keeping a journal, 45–46

Sleep — cont'd
    medications, 101, 103, 104
    naps, 104
    and pseudoephedrine, 103
    stages of, 102
    and stress, 90
Slouching posture, 64
SMART goals, 47–52
    maintaining goals, 151–153
Smoking
    how to quit, 112–114
    nicotine withdrawal, 113
SOLVE strategy, 90–91
Spinal cord
    role in pain signals, 3–4
Spinal nerve block, 130
Spirituality, 117–118
Steroid injections, 130
Strength, loss of, 27
Strength exercises, 60–63
Stress
    pain-stress cycle, 87
    physical response, 87–88
    reducing stress, 89–91
    relaxation, 91–94
    triggers, 88–89
Stretching, 56–58
Substance P, 4
Support groups, 155–156
Swayback posture, 64
Sympathetic nerve block, 130

T
Tai Chi, 140–141
Task modification, 71–72
Temperature extremes, 76
Temporomandibular joint disorders,
    20–21

Tension headache, 16
Thalamus, 4–5
Therapeutic touch, 141
Thumb flexibility exercises, 55
Tic douloureux, 20
Time management, 68–71, 89
TMJ. *See* Temporomandibular joint
    disorders
Trager, 138
Transcutaneous electric nerve
    stimulation (TENS), 141
Tricyclic antidepressants, 125–126
Trigeminal neuralgia, 20
Trigger-point injections, 130, 132
Trunk flexibility exercises, 56

V
Vasoconstrictors, 127

W
Walking, 59
Water aerobics, 59
Weight control, 104–108
    body mass index, 105–106
    losing weight, 107–108
Weight gain, 35–36
Weight lifting, 59, 60
Withdrawal (drug), 40, 124
Work issues, 38
    assertiveness, 84–85
    goal setting, 47–48, 51
World Wide Web information, 43
    Mayo Clinic Health Oasis, 129
Wrist flexibility exercises, 55

Y
Yoga, 136

MAYO CLINIC ON HEALTH

Arthritis

Chronic Pain

Depression

Digestive Health

Healthy Aging

Healthy Weight

High Blood Pressure

Managing Diabetes

Prostate Health

Vision

COMPACT GUIDES TO FITNESS AND HEALTH